Virtual Art Therapy

This book provides a practical and research-based exploration of virtual art psychotherapy, and how its innovations are breaking new ground in the mental health field.

With seventeen chapters authored by leaders documenting their research on creative arts therapies online, along with findings from the Virtual Art Therapy Clinic, this volume presents examples, strategies, and experiences delivering arts-based therapeutic services and online education. Clinical practice examples support and provide evidence for the transition from in-person to virtual sessions.

By combining the collected expertise of all the contributing authors, this book encourages art therapists to support further growth in the field of virtual art therapy.

Michelle Winkel is an art therapist, trained facilitator, and supervisor with twenty-five years of experience working directly with groups, families, and individuals. Michelle has taught art therapy at Loyola Marymount University in Los Angeles, IPATT in Bangkok, JIPATT in Tokyo, and VATI in Vancouver. As a supervisor at a local school agency in California for five years, she co-designed and implemented a reflective practice program that worked with the Child Protective Agency and other agencies in the area to improve supervision, performance, and morale of front-line staff. As a consultant, Michelle has used art therapy with businesses and organizations in group settings to improve organizational dynamics. Michelle, together with Dr. Maxine Junge, authored Graphic Facilitation and Art Therapy. Michelle's credentials include a license as a Marriage and Family Therapist in California and Registered Art Therapist in North America as well as a Registered Canadian Art Therapist. From 2004-2005, she held a fellowship in Infant-Parent Mental Health from Harvard Children's Hospital.

Virtual Art Therapy

Research and Practice

**Edited by
Michelle Winkel With Editorial
Assistance from Christel Bodenbender
and Melissa Yue**

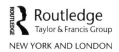

Routledge
Taylor & Francis Group

NEW YORK AND LONDON

Cover image by Cat Park

First published 2022
by Routledge
605 Third Avenue, New York, NY 10158

and by Routledge
4 Park Square, Milton Park, Abingdon, Oxon OX14 4RN

Routledge is an imprint of the Taylor & Francis Group, an informa business

Library of Congress Cataloging-in-Publication Data
A catalog record for this title has been requested

ISBN: 978-0-367-71152-8 (hbk)
ISBN: 978-0-367-71151-1 (pbk)
ISBN: 978-1-003-14953-8 (ebk)

DOI: 10.4324/9781003149538

Typeset in Times New Roman
by Taylor & Francis Books

To the Traveling Gals, Cheryl-Ann and Lauren

Contents

Figures

Tables

List of Contributors

Aditi Kaul, MA
Chapter 10: Squaring the Schaverien Triangle
Professional Art Therapist
UNESCO – CID Grade 5 certified Dance Movement Therapist
Programme lead, Expressive Arts Based Therapy pan-India
Department of Mental Health & Behavioral Sciences
Fortis Healthcare

Amber L. Cromwell, LMFT, ATR-BC
Chapter 6: Reaching City Youth with an Online Summer Arts Workshop in Los Angeles
Loyola Marymount University
Clinical supervisor in Helen B Landgarten Art Therapy Clinic
Director of Summer Arts Workshop
School-based counselor, Share & Care program
Cedars Sinai Medical Center

Ashley Nelson, BA
Chapter 4: Borders and Boundaries in Virtual Art Therapy
CiiAT – Canadian International Institute of Art Therapy
Diploma student
Virtual Art Therapy Clinic student therapist

Carolyn Brown Treadon, PhD, ATR-BC, ATCS
Chapter 11: Evolution of a Virtual Art Therapy Open Studio
Edinboro University
Graduate Program director, Art Therapy
Assistant professor
Department of Counseling, School Psychology, and Special Education

Christel Bodenbender, MA, CertAT
Editor
Chapter 15: Reducing Anxiety Levels during a Pandemic with Virtual Art Therapy: A Quasi-Experimental Pilot Study
Chapter 16: Art Therapy with Virtual Reality
Professional Art Therapist
CiiAT – Canadian International Institute of Art Therapy
Program and research coordinator

Girija Kaimal, EdD, MA, ATR-BC
Chapter 4: Borders and Boundaries in Virtual Art Therapy
Chapter 16: Art Therapy with Virtual Reality
Drexel University
Associate professor, PhD Program in Creative Arts Therapies
Assistant dean for Special Research Initiatives
Department of Creative Arts Therapies
President-elect, American Art Therapy Association (interviewee)

Gretchen M. Miller, MA, ATR-BC, ACTP
Chapter 17: Art Therapists and Digital Community
Director, American Art Therapy Association
Honorary life member, Buckeye Art Therapy Association
Adjunct faculty, Ursuline College Counseling and Art Therapy

Haley Toll, CCC, RCAT, RP (inactive)
Chapter 15: Reducing Anxiety Levels during a Pandemic with Virtual Art Therapy: A Quasi-Experimental Pilot Study
Memorial University of Newfoundland
Faculty of Education
PhD candidate

Hedaya AlDaleel, BFA, DCiiAT
Chapter 15: Reducing Anxiety Levels during a Pandemic with Virtual Art Therapy: A Quasi-Experimental Pilot Study
Professional Art Therapist
CiiAT – The Canadian International Institute of Art Therapy
Head of Student Services, Enrollment Department

Irit Hacmun, BA, MA
Chapter 16: Art Therapy with Virtual Reality
University of Haifa
Faculty of Social Welfare and Health Sciences, School of Creative Arts Therapies
(interviewee)

Iva Fattorini, MD, MSc
Chapter: Foreword
Founder, Artocene
Former chair & founder, Cleveland Clinic Arts & Medicine Institute
(interviewee)

Jessica Bianchi, EdD, ATR-BC, LMFT
Chapter 6: Reaching City Youth with an Online Summer Arts Workshop in Los Angeles
Loyola Marymount University
Assistant professor
Clinical director, Helen B. Landgarten Art Therapy Clinic
Department of Marital and Family Therapy with Specialization in Art Therapy

Jessica A. Walters
Chapter 3: Online Art Therapy: Experiences of Art Therapists During the COVID-19 Pandemic
School of the Art Institute of Chicago
Graduate assistant
Masters in Art Therapy and Counseling candidate

Jo Patcharin Sughondhabirom, MD, RCAT
Chapter 14: Online Art Therapy Classroom in Thailand
Coordinator, IPATT: International Program of Art Therapy in Thailand

Kate Collie, MA, MFA, PhD, ATR
Chapter 2: The Early Days of Online Art Therapy
Chapter 8: Keeping Up with the Times: Art Therapy Moves from Studio to Chat Room to Zoom
University of Alberta & Cross Cancer Institute
Assistant professor & clinical psychologist (retired)
Kickstart Disability Arts & Culture Board
Arts & Health researcher/developer

Kathryn Snyder, MA, ATR-BC, LPC
Chapter 5: Virtual Art Therapy with Children, Teens, and Families: A New Framework for Clinical Practice
Drexel University
Department of Creative Arts Therapies
PhD candidate

Lucille Proulx, MA, ATR, RCAT
Chapter 10: Squaring the Schaverien Triangle
CiiAT – The Canadian International Institute of Art Therapy
Director emeritus

Margaret Carlock-Russo, EdD, LCAT, ATR-BC, ATCS
Chapter 9: Reaching Older Adults through Virtual Art Therapy
Prescott College
Associate faculty and coordinator
Expressive Art Therapy Post Graduate Certificate Program
President, American Art Therapy Association

Marilyn Hahn, BEd, DCiiAT
Chapter 10: Squaring the Schaverien Triangle
Professional Art Therapist
Private practice art therapist and founder: Metamorph, Oh Sis!
Instructor, CiiAT – The Canadian International Institute of Art Therapy

Melissa Yue, BA
Editor
CiiAT – The Canadian International Institute of Art Therapy
Executive Assistant

Michele D. Rattigan, MA, ATR-BC, NCC, LPC
Chapter 12: Cameras Off, Coffee On: Online Teaching and Learning in COVID Times
Drexel University
College of Nursing & Health Professions
Clinical associate professor
Creative Arts Therapies Department
Graduate Art Therapy and Counseling Program

Michelle Winkel, MA, ATR, RCAT, REAT, MFT
Editor
Chapter 1: Our Changing Role: Expanding the Reach of Art Therapy
Chapter 4: Borders and Boundaries in Virtual Art Therapy
Chapter 13: Integrating Art Therapy with Nature-Based Practices
Chapter 15: Reducing Anxiety Levels during a Pandemic with Virtual Art Therapy: A Quasi-Experimental Pilot Study
CiiAT – The Canadian International Institute of Art Therapy
Clinical and academic director
Secretary, The Proulx Global Education and Community Foundation

Nicola Shaw, BA, PGCE, DCAT
Chapter 13: Integrating Art Therapy with Nature-Based Practices
Professional member of Canadian Art Therapy Association and the European Federation of Art Therapy
Founder of heartnature: stewardship & healing
Instructor, CiiAT – The Canadian International Institute of Art Therapy

Pamela Whitaker, PhD
Chapter 13: Integrating Art Therapy with Nature-Based Practices
Ulster University, Belfast School of Art
Course director, MSc Art Psychotherapy
Professional member of the British Association of Art Therapists and Irish Association of Creative Arts Therapists
Registered with Health and Care Professions Council (UK)
Fellow of the Higher Education Academy (UK)

Ronen Berger, PhD
Chapter 7: The Screen as a Stage: Artistic Methods for Group Arts-Based Therapy via Zoom
Ono Academic College
Head of the Drama Therapy MA Program
Instructor at Tel-Hai College
Founder of Nature Therapy

Sara Prins Hankinson, DVATI, RCAT
Chapter 8: Keeping Up With the Times: Art Therapy Moves from Studio to Chat Room to Zoom
Art therapist, BC Cancer Society
Supportive Cancer Department

Sheila Lorenzo de la Peña, PhD, ATR-BC, ATCS
Chapter 11: Evolution of a Virtual Art Therapy Open Studio
Edinboro University
Assistant professor in Art Therapy
Department of Counseling, School Psychology, and Special Education
Art Therapy Undergraduate Program director

Valerie Behiery, BFA, MA, PhD, DCiiAT
Chapter 4: Borders and Boundaries in Virtual Art Therapy
Professional Art Therapist
Al Faisal University
Assistant professor
Department of Humanities and Social Sciences

Acknowledgements

I would like to thank Cheryl-Ann Webster for her unending support of my endeavours, including this project. From this book's inception, when Lucille Proulx, Cheryl-Ann, and I gathered in Lucille's backyard sharing our learnings about virtual art therapy early in 2020, she was encouraging, visionary, and strategic. She knew that the time I needed to complete this ambitious project would impact her and our organization, so thank you! To my editorial team, Melissa Yue and Christel Bodenbender, thank you for your persistence, skill, humour, and commitment. Melissa is a fiction writer, and Christel is a speculative fiction writer and art therapist, so the calibre of technical and content support was always high. They both made the process fun and focused.

To the authors, thank you for sharing your knowledge and creativity which makes this book possible!

To the students providing art therapy in our virtual clinic, thank you for pioneering new ways of interacting with clients, helping troubleshoot technical challenges, and your dedication to providing innovative methodologies from week to week.

To the clients we serve, thank you for sharing your wisdom and vulnerabilities with your student therapists and their supervisors. This continues to be the reason we are art therapists, and the relationships with you fuel us.

To the rest of the CiiAT team, including Lucille Proulx and Behan Webster, I am so grateful for your support and expertise at every turn.

To my family, Tonya, Jamie, Mom and Dad, and to my wife, Lauren Nackman, who was an important part of the editorial team and is always my tireless cheerleader.

Foreword

Iva Fattorini

When I present to people who know nothing about art therapy, I begin to describe it but often move directly into an intervention that I was taught by an art therapy colleague. I ask them to take a pencil and paper, and to think about how their day was and to simply draw a line without saying anything. Then I ask them how their week went and draw the line, and then I ask them how was their month, and how was their year, and their life. People are always profoundly moved. Only then do they realize the power of nonverbal expression. In those moments of reflection, in silence, when they were drawing one line—their whole life in one line—one pencil mark. Imagine adding colours and shapes, and oil pastels or paint or sculpting materials. Then add a guide in this process; a witness to the unfolding process: the art therapist.

The articles presented in this volume provide the keys to making the paradigm shift that I believe is necessary by showing the strengths of art therapy, and especially virtual art therapy, as a way to add value to contemporary medical care. Although I am a physician and not an art therapist, I was humbled and grateful to be able to learn from the art therapists with whom I worked while establishing the Cleveland Clinic Arts & Medicine Institute. I witnessed art therapists working very closely with their patients and realized that in hospital settings, art is not a commodity, it's a necessity. A hospital experience that includes the arts has a profound impact on patients, families and caregivers.

I often ask myself when the world will prioritize emotional and mental health. It's a problem that we continuously ignore—perhaps because in a world driven by hard data, it is not easy to quantify the impact of therapy. My hope is that when we can prove that art therapy lowers the cost in healthcare and improves mental health, it will be more accepted and more highly regarded. An integration of all forms of arts and creative expression therapies to healthcare increases the level of humanity in healthcare and transforms it to better care for patients beyond science alone.

Art therapy is not a soft and fuzzy intervention. It's not just playing with materials; it is a profound process involving our deepest emotions, connecting us with the areas of the brain that we can't access with speech. It allows us to be able to express ourselves through other avenues. Thus, significant change can occur using art therapy as part of prevention in healthcare. We must try to lower the chance of mental health issues by starting at an early age, when most mental health concerns begin.

In medicine, decisions are based on evidence. Many studies conducted around the integration of arts and medicine have demonstrated improvements in health outcomes, quality of life, and improved hospital experiences. Increasingly, more research is becoming available about the effectiveness of art therapy, as well as studies demonstrating the effectiveness of telehealth and tele-mental health. However, research on virtual art therapy is in its infancy, which is why this book is critical and timely. We must commit to continued research on the value of art therapy, the applications of virtual treatment modalities to provide more client options, and the development of the evidence that is so important to establish credibility for the field. I believe that, as we find in this volume, both hard research and humanizing stories are needed to establish credibility.

I believe nothing can replace personal human contact and creating tactile art, but the COVID-19 pandemic has forced us to think differently. As a proponent of digital technologies to increase accessibility for clients and patients to art therapy, I believe art therapists are extremely brave for embracing these new technologies and techniques in order to respond quickly during the pandemic. As you read the stories of the authors, and those of their clients and students, I hope you will feel inspired by their bravery and innovation.

1 Our Changing Role

Expanding the Reach of Art Therapy

Michelle Winkel

Recent pressures around the world due to physical distance, along with increasing access to low-cost internet services and equipment, make conducting art therapy over online platforms a viable and important option. One of the most pressing issues with in-person therapy is often the lack of access for populations who need therapeutic services the most. Single parents may not be able to leave their homes to attend weekly appointments. Youth might struggle finding safe transportation to go to a therapist's office. Ageing seniors may not be aware of therapy options within their community. Despite the world becoming more connected over the last decades, we are, in many ways, failing to connect with the most vulnerable populations. As a growing number of art therapists become confident and competent in providing online, or *virtual*, art therapy, it is our sincere hope that more clients will benefit from this development worldwide. Throughout this book, we propose that the best of in-person art therapy can be safely transferred to virtual platforms in order to expand its reach to a much wider population.

In general, clinical and counselling psychology services are inequitably distributed, with shortages in remote and rural areas of most countries (Simpson & Reid, 2014). The outreach possibility of virtual art therapy helps extend the access of services to isolated and marginalized people, including:

- Rural and remote populations
- Populations reluctant to leave their homes, including the growing number of people struggling with anxiety, agoraphobia, and social phobias
- Persons not comfortable going outside the home for traditional psychotherapy in cultures that stigmatize mental health practices
- Persons required to stay physically distant due to health considerations
- Confined populations
- Persons who do not have the time to commute or are most comfortable online
- Disabled or differently abled populations who are unable to physically access outside therapy services
- Military personnel

Virtual art therapy can provide a critical alternative for these populations, including people like Wayne Smith[1].

DOI: 10.4324/9781003149538-1

Wayne is a military veteran who has served several tours of duty. After retiring, he moved with his family to a farming community without a registered art therapist. He deals well with balancing his physical pain from injuries sustained in service, and emotional challenges related to PTSD. While he doesn't identify as an artist, he finds joy in making marks, painting, and drawing shapes on big sheets of cardboard, and is able to access art therapy services through our online clinic. His therapist acts as a witness to his newly discovered creative process and joins him in co-creating a more pleasurable day-to-day life.

A note about terminology: 'Virtual' is the term used in this book for synchronous online videoconferencing, in which the therapist and client can see each other simultaneously through a webcam, and hear each other through the computer microphones or telephone. It is a generic term that does not distinguish between web conferencing platforms such as Zoom, Microsoft Teams, Jane, Doxy, SharePoint, and others. In this context, tel-etherapy pioneer Kate Collie chronicles the early days of telehealth and art therapy in Chapter 2, discussing videoconferencing predecessors, which includes other forms of electronic communication, such as tele-phone, email, text, fax, chat, forums, that have been—and in some cases continue—to be used.

Fundamentals Are Still Fundamental: Ethics, Security, Confidentiality

The fundamentals of art therapy have not changed; the art therapist working virtually is responsible for gaining informed consent, sharing the limits of confidentiality, and conveying in clear language the potential risks of working online. As in face-to-face therapy, the art therapist conducts a thorough intake and initial assessment to determine if there is a therapeutic fit, including the client's suitability and capacity for working remotely. For example, most cli-ents in immediate crisis or clients who struggle with orientation to reality or have significant trauma usually need to be referred to a local service provider in their area. Helping support the client to make those linkages falls within this practice. Next, the art therapist collaboratively guides the process of establishing treatment goals based on the client's presenting challenges and experiences. Helping the client to create a virtual studio for art making and dialoguing with the client about the creative process and their artwork con-tinue to be focal points in virtual art therapy. Therapists must also adhere to relevant privacy legislation and counselling regulatory bodies, which vary depending on where the art therapist resides and works. Issues of security must be addressed with the client, such as encryption of the video platform, firewalls, and anti-virus and anti-malware software, and how this might impact the client's personal information (Le Bihan, 2020). Therapists should also implement and inform clients about their policies and procedures concerning the safe storage, transfer, and disposal of data. Insurance coverage across provincial and national boundaries, which is continually shifting, remains the responsibility of the therapist. While many issues are similar to the brick-and-mortar art therapy studio, working virtually does require extra training, knowledge, and equipment—the art therapist's task. In a recent UK-wide survey about online art therapy practice and client safety, therapists' confidence was found to be generally lower with respect to providing online art therapy sessions in relation to in-person therapy (Zubala & Hackett, 2020). We aim to change that for our readers.

The Therapeutic Alliance: Same Glue, Different Container

When you think of effective art therapy, what comes to mind? Perhaps it's a client's subjective view of their progress, or a certain level of trust between that client and their therapist—in other words, the therapeutic alliance. The therapeutic alliance, or working alliance, is often considered the cornerstone for successful outcomes in many therapies (Doran, 2016), including art therapy. It can be summarized as the affective bond or attachment between therapist and client, the collaborative quality of the relationship, and the ability of the therapist and client to agree on mutually acceptable therapeutic tasks and goals (Simpson & Reid, 2014). A solid therapeutic alliance is a connection unlike any other.

When clients are physically separated from their therapists through communication tools such as videoconferencing, the therapist may be concerned about the development of the therapeutic alliance. The loss of ability to see the client, their artwork, and the process of creating that artwork in one physical space may be uncomfortable. In the tele-mental health field, however, various research studies conclude that the therapeutic alliance is not negatively impacted by telecommunication tools (Wehmann et al., 2020). Themes from this prior research suggest that clients often show lessened inhibitions to disclose intimate details about their lives when conducting therapy through technological aids (Beyens et al., 2018). Authors AlDaleel, Proulx, and Sughondhabirom will share their observations of reduced inhibition in students and clients during online art therapy and education when compared with in-person art therapy in Chapters 4, 10, and 11.

Jerome and Zaylor (2000) first identified several differences between in-person and online therapies, including a slower rate of communication, differences in depth perception, and interpersonal distance. Despite these differences, they found that videoconferencing's unique factors may actually enhance some psychotherapeutic endeavours. For example, videoconferencing requires turn-taking—a skill that some clients need to practice in therapy—as both participants cannot be heard at the same time. Clients in videoconferencing sessions must also engage in additional awareness of what the other participant can see, particularly if they are switching between views of themselves and views of their art making. Skills acquired during these online sessions can be immediately practiced in daily lives. Many of our authors explore these differences and include vignettes to convey their findings.

It is understandable, however, that some art therapists have been hesitant to take their professional practice online. Studies undertaken in Australia with psychologists indicate that they were concerned that the therapist would be compromised in being able to communicate warmth, understanding, sensitivity, and empathy as a result of the video medium (Rees & Stone, 2005). Despite numerous studies rebutting this, the negative bias persists. One of the goals of this book is to ease the sense of discomfort or belief that virtual art therapy is less valuable than in-person therapy. Indeed, there are logistical, ethical, and technical challenges that must be carefully considered. This book addresses and explores these challenges, shares new discoveries, current research, as well as new practice concepts and techniques to inspire our readers.

Shifting the Power Balance

As with in-person therapy, virtual art therapy starts with building trust between the client and the therapist. A successful beginning entails helping the client value their creative process and involves the supportive and clear boundaries of the therapist to guide the initial process. For art therapy to be productive for the client with the challenges that brought them to therapy, it is essential to create something meaningful and authentic in the therapeutic alliance. Conducting sessions through videoconferencing requires a different level of effort to create an atmosphere of trust (Le Bihan, 2020). Technological issues may also cause interference. Low bandwidth can cause audio lags or visual distortions. It is important for the therapist to feel competent in guiding the client to technical solutions and have alternatives and backup plans in place. Throughout this book, authors share their innovative solutions to technological and ethical challenges.

In a traditional setting, the therapist's studio or office is the familiar, safe, and containing space that the client regularly visits. In virtual art therapy, the therapist has considerably less control over the physical space of the client. They are essentially visiting the client in their home or wherever they choose to be sitting for their sessions. The client is now the designer and holder of their own physical therapeutic space and will need guidance from the art therapist on how to turn that space into a suitable environment that they can associate with positive, creative, and healing work. In the virtual relationship, both client and therapist are responsible for safety and privacy (Weinberg & Rolnick, 2020).

Hanaa is in her mid-30s and deals with symptoms of anxiety. She has been doing online art therapy through the Virtual Art Therapy Clinic at the Canadian International Institute of Art Therapy for a few months. She says,

"There is the benefit of using my own tools and supplies. There is a comfort that comes from using what I own that I don't think I recognized before. There is a relationship built between myself and those objects ... a healthy, healing relationship that extends far beyond the one-hour session. And lastly, the inner strength that I build within a session transcends into my everyday life much faster, as opposed to leaving my strong self in the therapy office to return to that person only at my next appointment."

"I have had years of experience with psychotherapy, from talk therapy to somatic experiencing. I have processed a lot of painful traumatic experiences through these therapies, and I am very grateful for them. However, art therapy has been a completely new and powerful experience for me. A completely liberating experience."

In art therapy, one of the goals for the client is to discover new and unexpected outcomes through the art making process. This vital process can only happen based on a strong relationship with the therapist. The image, picture, video, collage, or sculpture that the client makes in art therapy becomes a third element, and creates the therapeutic relationship triangle (Schaverien, 1999). In the triangular relationship, two sets of eyes look together at the art piece in joint attention. This process of joint attention prioritizes the art as a piece of value in its own right, causing it to almost function as a third entity in the therapeutic dynamic (Isserow, 2008). In virtual art therapy, we propose that there is a fourth element: the computer screen. We call it "Squaring the Schaverien Triangle" and will explore this in Chapter 10.

Setting up the Studio and Other Practical Considerations

As the physical space is no longer determined solely by the art therapist, they should offer to help the client set up their studio. They will need to brainstorm together where to store the artwork the client creates so that it is kept protected from family members, pets, or others. This includes digital storage in encrypted, password-protected devices. Maybe the client lives with several family members and does not have a room with a door that closes and therefore may not have the sense of privacy that the therapist feels is best practice. These considerations will give rise to additional negotiations that should be instigated by the art therapist. For example, there may be certain times of the day that the client has privacy in their home.

One of our clients, who we will call Sanjana, took several sessions to settle into a routine and space that worked for her. For the first few weeks, her therapist noted that Sanjana was in a new room every session. She was disorganized with her art supplies and seemed unsettled in her space. In a sensitive manner, her art therapist commented on what she observed. "What is your favourite room, Sanjana?" Sanjana replied, "The one I was in the first week, but my husband uses that room sometimes. He's in there now, so I can't be in there today."

Together, they discussed alternatives and worked out days and times for their next sessions. They decided to have appointments when Sanjana's husband was typically sleeping. That way, she could be in her favourite room for sessions, claiming, both literally and symbolically, a private space she rarely has in her home. The art therapist also invited her to bring special objects and mementos gathered from dusty corners of the house into that room as an act of nurturance. This small action became a positive step in Sanjana's healing journey.

A different client talked about being the "master of her own domain." She writes:

> Working online has been incredibly rewarding. If I rush through the obvious benefits of saving time through not commuting, not having the stress of navigating traffic, and saving parking fees, there are other deeper, unexpected benefits that I have experienced. I am in my own space. There is no need to enter a therapy office and feel like a patient, which happens regardless of how comfortable or homelike the office may be. This has contributed to the truly collaborative relationship that I have built with my art therapist. I am the "master of my own domain", and I believe this brings a strength to the work that I would not have had otherwise.

If the client does not have the resources to purchase art materials, the therapist can help them choose alternative media that are readily accessible in their environment. Sand, leaves, and sticks from their local garden might be brought to the next session. Curious, found objects may be hiding in their closet, such as keys, glasses, boxes, string, or recycled bottles. A look into the kitchen pantry might turn up food items like lentils, pasta, turmeric powder, and other tactile and sensory materials. Digital drawing tools might also be considered if the client has access to such programs.

It is important to note that virtual art therapy does not depend on digital art-making methods. Although it can encompass digital-based media and activities, it can also include many traditional and non-traditional art materials used by art therapists in face-to-face psychotherapy. The only exceptions are those materials the client cannot access. The client creates the artwork from materials they have on hand, and the ability to choose materials can give the client an added feeling of being in charge of their own therapeutic journey. They may choose emotionally charged items that allow them greater access to unconscious material and arrive more swiftly at resolutions of trauma or depression. Smelly, gooey clay, or wood shavings and carpenter's glue from a garage can stimulate childhood memories for some. Spontaneously recorded videos made with the art therapist during sessions can give immediate playback opportunities while tapping into previously inaccessible emotions. In our experience, the home environment is a blessing in disguise for the art therapist.

Although they are not able to wow their clients with an array of sensual art materials in their own studio—which can feel like a loss in the beginning of a therapeutic encounter—with skill and negotiation with the client, alternatives are sometimes more meaningful and unique to the client's own journey. Many of our authors explore media in their chapters, including video, playback theatre, painting, found objects, photography, the digital whiteboard, and virtual reality.

In summary, we believe that most of the curative factors in art therapy, including the therapeutic alliance, as well as the use of art making with both traditional and non-traditional media, can be transferred to online platforms. How we incorporate these factors will depend largely on what is accessible, and, perhaps more importantly, how we view our rapidly changing technological modalities. Ethical considerations are paramount, and it is the art therapists' responsibility to educate themselves through ongoing training and supervision, and for art therapy training programs to be the leaders in virtual art therapy practice, and research.

Another client, Sam, talks about her experience of closeness with her therapist in virtual art therapy.

Art therapy has been a tool which has allowed me to express what my unconscious mind always wanted to say … and I believe, always wanted to let go of … and all without words; this has been amazing to me. The relationship I have had with my art therapist has been quite different from my other therapists. Instead of looking to my art therapist as the holder of all wisdom and solutions, she has been my guide to discovering my own wisdom and solutions. It's a wholeness that I have never felt before, regardless of the extreme talent of my past therapists. It's a self-trust, a self-compassion that I have never experienced in any other therapeutic relationship, perhaps because my unconsciousness is also part of this triad. I can feel my art therapist's strength and confidence in my own healing power. She introduces me to my own inner self. Perhaps this has been my biggest learning from virtual art therapy.

Book Sections and Themes Overview

This diverse collection of chapters is organized into sections by theme. Section 1 "How Did We Get Here?" gives us a foundation for what we currently call *virtual art therapy*. It starts in Chapter 2 with Collie's review of the past two decades of distance art therapy in its earlier forms. Many of the discoveries about what works for clients comes from the work of these early researchers and practitioners. Ultimately, technology is not therapy—the therapeutic relationship is still central (Agar, 2020). Next, Walters (Chapter 3) summarizes her study findings on the

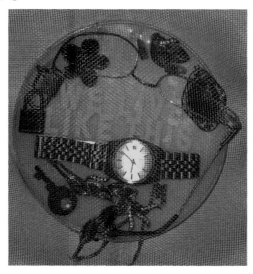

Figure 1.1 Household Found Objects, Created by Client "Maria"

experiences of art therapists navigating the sudden leap to online art therapy in 2020. This study highlights the themes and challenges of this work, motifs which come up throughout subsequent chapters and prepare the reader for the landscape.

The following Section 2 "Clinical Perspectives" draws on the authors' experiments with various populations, essentially trials-by-fire brought on by global physical distancing mandates. While some authors had experience working virtually before the pandemic, clients no longer had the choice to visit their therapists face-to-face, causing an urgency and air of innovation that readers will witness in these chapters. In this section, each author discovers their unique solutions to best practice with specific populations.

When working with seniors, for example, Carlock-Russo (Chapter 9) dis-covered that bringing caregivers into the art therapy work not only helped clients navigate the virtual session space, assisted with setting up materials, and aided caregivers in their own stress relief, but their presence was essential to the effectiveness of art therapy. Ultimately, Carlock-Russo shifted sessions to dyadic practice, where it had once been individual therapy with seniors. Looking at a younger population, Bianchi and Cromwell (Chapter 6) worked with youth in the prison system, helping them identify their strengths through art making. The therapists displayed themselves in real time on video for the clients to see them, but due to security and legal restrictions, they could not see the clients. Innovating ways to foster the therapeutic relationship and keep the art central is the focus of their chapter.

In Chapter 4, through a dialogue with Kaimal, I share my learnings on working with diverse clients and students across borders in a virtual art therapy clinic. Changing art therapy approaches often entails online adaptation to existing methods. Snyder describes her discoveries with the 'magic circle' as a therapy space online in Chapter 5, working with children and families in new ways. Berger explores playback theatre when working with groups online in Chapter 7, "The screen as stage." He does not adapt a face-to-face practice into an online modality but forges an entirely new intervention. Hankinson and Collie (Chapter 8) write about their work with moving art therapy with cancer patients from studio to chat room to Zoom.

In Section 3 "Innovations in Training and Supervision", we discuss shifts in art therapy training programs and innovative curriculum designs. Focusing on art therapy supervision in Chapter 10, Proulx shares vignettes from supervisees working online in several countries. In Chapter 11, Treadon and de La Pena explore the historical roots of the open studio in art therapy, modern uses, Edinboro University's approach to a campus-based open studio, and the shift to a virtual platform following the closure of its community studio space. Going one step further, Rattigan (Chapter 12) deconstructs and rebuilds a course online and explores synchronous and asynchronous class elements, including a virtual art coffeehouse with students.

Chapter 14 describes collaborations in the online classroom in a training program in Bangkok, Thailand. A small student survey between in-person and online art therapy education revealed that the process of group formation was slower online than in-person. Author Sughondhabirom, however, also discovered the greater comfort of some students to show their vulnerability with classmates in an online setting compared to the usual in-person class setting.

In Chapter 15, we continue with a study on virtual art therapy and its effects on anxiety levels in clients. The study was carried out at the virtual art therapy clinic at the Canadian International Institute of Art Therapy, where student art therapists recorded their clients' anxiety levels before and after each session. Early findings suggest that remote art therapy sessions may be a suitable treatment modality for anxiety, particularly during the current pandemic.

Whittaker, Shaw, and I expand the art therapy studio in Chapter 13 into the outdoors in the form of walking studios and eco art therapy training, such as blogs, and shared online viewing of mock video sessions to train students in this alternative art therapy approach.

In the last section of this book, Section 4 "Virtual Vistas", Bodenbender, Kaimal, and Hacmun (Chapter 16) explore virtual reality and its emerging place in the field of art therapy, and Miller (Chapter 17) shares the time capsule she created within the digital art therapy community. While more research in this burgeoning field is an ongoing necessity, it is my hope that this book will provide you with new tools, confidence, and enthusiasm for augmenting your own practice with virtual art therapy.

Note

1 Please note that all names have been changed in this book for confidentiality purposes. All images used in this book have been included with explicit permission.

References

Agar, G. (2020). The clinic offers no advantage over the screen, for relationship is everything. In H. Weinberg & A. Rolnick (Eds.), *Theory and practice of online therapy: Internet-delivered interventions for individuals, groups, families, and organizations: Video psychotherapy and its dynamics* (pp. 66–78). Routledge.

Beyens, I., Valkenburg, P. M., & Piotrowski, J. T. (2018). Screen media use and ADHD-related behaviors: Four decades of research. *Proceedings of the National Academy of Sciences*, *115*(40), 9875–9881. https://doi.org/10.1073/pnas.1611611114.

Doran, J. M. (2016). The working alliance: Where have we been, where are we going? *Journal of the Society for Psychotherapy Research*, *26*(2), 146–163. https://doi.org/10.1080/10503307.2014.954153.

Isserow, J. (2008). Looking together: Joint attention in art therapy. *International Journal of Art Therapy*, *13*(1), 34–42. https://doi.org/10.1080/17454830802002894.

Jerome, L., & Zaylor, C. (2000). Cyberspace: Creating a therapeutic environment for telehealth applications. *Professional Psychology Research and Practice*, *31*(5), 478–483. https://doi.apa.org/doi/10.1037/0735-7028.31.5.478.

Le Bihan, N. (2020). *Guidelines for electronic practices in art therapy* [*Unpublished*]. Kutenai Art Therapy Institute.

Rees, C., & Stone, S. (2005). Therapeutic alliance in face-to-face versus videoconferenced psychotherapy. *Professional Psychology Research and Practice*, *36*(6), 649–653. https://doi.org/10.1037/0735-7028.31.5.478.

Schaverien, J. (1999). *The revealing image: Analytical art psychotherapy in theory and practice*. Jessica Kingsley Publishers.

Simpson, S. G., & Reid, C. L. (2014). Therapeutic alliance in videoconferencing psychotherapy: A review. *The Australian Journal of Rural Health*, *22*, 280–299. https://doi.org/10.1111/ajr.12149.

Wehmann, E., Köhnen, M., Härter, M., & Liebherz, S. (2020, June). Therapeutic alliance in technology-based interventions for the treatment of depression: Systematic review. *Journal of Medical Internet Research*, *22*(6), e17195. doi:10.2196/17195.

Weinberg, H., & Rolnick, A. (2020). Introduction. In H. Weinberg & A. Rolnick (Eds.), *Theory and practice of online therapy: Internet-delivered interventions for individuals, groups, families, and organizations* (pp. 1–10). Routledge.

Zubala, A., & Hackett, S. (2020). Online art therapy practice and client safety: A UK-wide survey in times of COVID-19. *International Journal of Art Therapy*, *25*(4), 161–171. https://doi.org/10.1080/17454832.2020.1845221.

Section I

How Did We Get Here?

2 The Early Days of Online Art Therapy

Kate Collie

Introduction

To see how online art therapy began, let's go back to the mid-1990s when the internet was just coming into its own. Across the industrialized world, people with computers were starting to turn to the World Wide Web for information and were starting to use the internet (always spelled with a capital 'I' back then) for email. If you had a computer and an internet service provider, you could pay to 'dial in' through your telephone landline if no one was using the telephone. It was awkward to juggle phone use and internet use. Cell phones existed, but hardly anyone had one. There were no smartphones. Long-distance telephone calls were uncommon because they were expensive. Bandwidth was limited. Anything from the internet had to go through tiny phone lines. This might be hard to imagine if you weren't alive then. If you were, it might be hard to remember how different it was.

Social media sites were barely beginning. An early site called Six Degrees was launched in 1997, but didn't last. LinkedIn began in 2002 and Facebook in 2004. Weblogs, or blogs, became popular in 1999. Google got its start in 1997 as a student research project and was incorporated in 1998 (Shah, 2016). This was the dot-com era when the value of technology companies was skyrocketing and venture capitalists were funding all manner of innovative ideas related to the internet.

It was a different world, but things were changing rapidly. There was excitement about using the internet for *telehealth*—a word coined to refer to the use of the internet and other telecommunications technologies to extend the reach of healthcare, including mental health services (often called behavioural health services), and to increase equality of access. This was especially true in Australia and Canada, two technologically advanced countries with populations spread across vast geographical distances with many rural and remote communities. Telecommunications technologies, such as telephones and radios, had been used in Canada to facilitate healthcare from a distance for many decades (Cervinkas, 1984). Hence, it was natural to begin utilizing the internet. People in Canada, Australia, and elsewhere began exploring online psychotherapy and counselling. It was only a matter of time until art therapy joined the online world.

DOI: 10.4324/9781003149538-3

Online Art Therapy Begins

By 1997, a few art therapists in Canada and Australia were offering asynchronous online art therapy using email with image attachments. They offered this to clients who lived far from any art therapist or who couldn't leave their homes for health reasons; for example, clients with AIDS, which was widespread at the time. Asynchronous communication, which entails a delayed response, such as with email, texting, or letter writing, can be contrasted with synchronous communication, where responses are immediate, such as with videoconferencing, phone calls, and in-person communication.

Controversy and Trepidation

The idea of offering counselling, psychotherapy, or art therapy via the internet was controversial. At a time before cell phones and videoconferencing platforms, clients and therapists would neither see nor hear each other during online therapy sessions. The lack of visual non-verbal cues was a great concern.

Some therapists argued that it would be unethical or flat-out impossible to do therapy without seeing their clients and therefore without access to non-verbal cues—not recognizing that non-verbal cues come in many forms, as Murphy and Mitchell demonstrated in their articles about email therapy (Murphy & Mitchell, 1998; Collie et al., 2000). In addition to the lack of visual cues, a range of other potential problems with online therapy were identified (Sampson et al., 1997), which included verifying the identity of the other person, protecting confidentiality and ensuring privacy, having adequate referral information for clients in different locations, dealing with technical failure, and dealing with differences in laws, payment structures, and standards of practice in the client's and therapist's locations. Equality of access to computers was another concern.

Potential benefits were described, too, in addition to expanded access to services, and included reduced power imbalances between clients and therapists, less likelihood of dependence on the therapist, a greater sense on the part of the client of being responsible for positive change, and the possibility of including family members in the therapeutic process. Overall, it was *therapists* who were skeptical about online therapy where they would not be able to see their clients, and *clients* who were in favour of online services where they would not have to be seen. It was a startling difference.

The possible benefits and risks of text-only online therapy that were being discussed at the time set the stage for ethical guidelines. The first set of ethical guidelines for online counselling was published in 1998 (Bloom), having been created by an international team of experts. Those early guidelines became a foundation for all future ethical considerations for distance psychotherapy, counselling, and art therapy.

Virtual House Call

Early proponents of telehealth, including tele-therapy, saw it as a way to a) improve access to healthcare while bringing down costs, b) increase availability of health and wellness information, and, most importantly, c) make healthcare available to groups that historically had been underserved, such as the elderly, people in rural and remote regions, marginalized people, and people with disabilities or mobility constraints. In spite of trepidations about safety and confidentiality, early research about telehealth was promising and created the idea of a 'virtual house call,' where the client could stay at home and health services they needed would come to them by way of the internet. Imagine what this meant to someone who had been travelling many hours to attend medical appointments, or to anyone so ill that leaving home to get care could be more harmful than helpful, especially if there would be hours spent in waiting rooms. Imagine how excited medical professionals were at the thought of reaching people in remote areas who otherwise had no access to specialized health services.

Video conferencing

Hospitals started purchasing expensive videoconferencing equipment for communication between hospitals and special high-bandwidth lines were installed between medical facilities. Videoconferencing was so impressive (and costly!) at the beginning that it got much of the telehealth attention, even though the quality was poor. Often the audio and video were not synchronized. Videoconferencing, however, was not an option for individuals or small organizations and the prohibitive cost went against the goal of expanding access to healthcare and making more equitable use of available monetary resources. Affordable options were needed, as were ways to cover the 'last mile'—the distance between a hospital or clinic with telehealth equipment and a person's home. This was difficult because of bandwidth constraints at the time.

The types of inexpensive video communication we use now did not exist. Skype didn't start until 2003 and Zoom did not appear until 2011. Video telephones had been on the market briefly in the 1970s (Picturephones by AT&T), but consumer interest was low for something that made telephones feel less private. Attitudes toward privacy and telephones, however, have changed dramatically since then. Ironically, it might be low-bandwidth forms of teletherapy that solve a present-day problem with privacy in online art therapy, which is that clients might not have a private enough place for art therapy using a video communication platform, such as Zoom, and may opt for text or email.

Advantages of Technologically Mediated Communication

Throughout the 1990s, research was conducted across multiple domains to determine the pros and cons of *mediated communication* (communication from a distance using telecommunications technologies) to help understand the potential of the internet. In fields such as social psychology and special education, people wanted to know how interpersonal communication differs when people are in the same location or not, whether they can be seen or just heard, and so on. This resulted in a fascinating body of research, much of it published around 1996, that helped shape early forms of online art therapy.

There were comparisons between in-person communication, where you hear and see a person who is with you; to telephoning, where you hear a person you don't see; face-to-face videoconferencing, where you hear and see a person who is not with you; and communication where you don't see each other but look at something together, such as a whiteboard in the business world, or artwork in online art therapy. Synchronous communication in real time was compared with asynchronous communication where responses are delayed, such as with email. Speech communication was compared with writing and typing. Researchers measured such things as effectiveness of communication, speed of task completion, task focus, honesty, trust development, relationship formation, intimacy, and willingness to communicate (see Collie, 2004 for a summary).

Surprising Results

One of the biggest insights that researchers discovered was that it was hard to find significant differences between types of communication. Humans are such flexible communicators that we take whatever mode of communication is available to us and adapt it to our needs, especially for relationship formation and emotional closeness. *Social information processing* theory (Walther, 1992) explains that people using any communication medium experience similar needs for uncertainty reduction and affinity, and adapt their ways of communicating over time to favour "the solicitation and presentation of socially revealing, relational behaviour" (Walther et al., 1994, p. 465). Hence, in order to meet these needs, people do not let the communication medium stand in the way, especially when the medium favours nuanced communication (Robertson, 1997). This doesn't mean that all modes of communication are equivalent. Rather, it means that each one has its strengths. Art therapists offering art therapy from a distance can benefit from knowing about these strengths, especially for situations where video communication is not an option. Several such situations are discussed in the chapters of this book.

Why Mediated Communication is Sometimes Better

Walther (1996) coined the term *hyperpersonal communication* to describe no-sight mediated communication that enhances social and emotional communication beyond what usually happens in face-to-face communication. Walther stated that even text-only communication can sometimes be more intimate and socially oriented than face-to-face communication because of (a) *idealization*, which is the tendency for people to inflate their perceptions of people they do not see by using the few social cues they have to create a positive image of the person with whom they are communicating; (b) the possibility for people to *optimize their self-presentations* by being selective about what they reveal, especially early on; (c) the fact that *more attention* can be devoted to the communication when attention is not being used for the intricacies of a face-to-face social interaction; and (d) the possibility of what he calls an *intensification loop* of positive reciprocation, whereby people who are addressed as if they are attractive and socially desirable (because of being invisible) will tend to behave that way.

Weinberg (1996) found that an absence of visual cues had an enhancing effect on mediated communication in her study of perceived supportiveness. Other researchers found that people feel less vulnerable and more free to speak when they cannot be seen (Fish, 1990; Graetz et al., 1998). Citera (1998) found that less dominating people were more able to influence decisions when communicating by telephone or text.

When there are no visual cues from facial expressions, people tend to compensate with speech, especially when checking for understanding. Doherty-Sneddon et al. (1997) found that even with videoconferencing that made it possible to see eye movements and other fine-grained visual cues that are used in in-person communication, their research participants continued to check for understanding verbally. In this way, they used cognitive effort to communicate both as if they were together and as if they were not together at the same time. Doherty-Sneddon et al. coined the term 'over-gazing' to refer to this doubling of effort and speculated that people thought they would be able to use visual signals in the same way as in face-to-face communication, attempted to do this, but found it difficult to trust visual cues from videoconferencing. Doherty-Sneddon et al. concluded that what we think of as visual cues are probably not solely visual. They, among others, have shown that videoconferencing can take more cognitive processing than it is worth. During videoconferencing sessions, visual information about people and their settings will be viewed, processed, and evaluated over and over again, even if the information stays the same minute after minute and nothing new is added (Doherty-Sneddon et al., 1997; Sproull & Kiesler, 1996). This takes cognitive effort and can be tiring. Sproull and Kiesler (1996) found that in no-sight communication, when it is not necessary to monitor the other person's visual and social cues, attention can be freed up for focusing on the communication tasks at hand. In online art therapy, a task might be listening with empathy. Colòn (1999) also found that task focus increased in no-sight encounters when there were fewer visual distractions and less concern about social appearances.

Mediated Communication and Behavioural Telehealth

In mediated communication research, specifically about psychotherapy, counselling, and other forms of psychosocial support, no-sight communication was similar to in-person communication on most measures, especially if there was initial face-to-face contact. Preliminary studies of mediated communication for psychiatric consultations (Ball et al., 1995; Yellowlees & Kennedy, 1996), brief psychotherapy (Day & Schneider, 2000), and counselling (Cohen & Kerr, 1998) found no significant differences between audio, video, and in-person modes of communication on measures such as relationship formation, therapeutic outcomes, and client satisfaction. The potential for successful distance mental health services was claimed more-or-less equally for all forms of communication, although with telephone and online services, stronger claims could be made about reaching hard-to-reach people (Zhu et al., 1996).

Human Factors Matter Most

As behavioural telehealth research accumulated, it seemed that the success of the particular telehealth service would depend less on what type of communication technology was used and more on *how* it was used (Stamm, 1998; Yellowlees & Kennedy, 1996). With the rise of the internet and the appearance of many new telecommunications technologies during the dot-com era, there was a tendency to focus on the technologies themselves rather than on what they were for. For example, when we developed technology for online art therapy in the late 1990s, it was sometimes hard to explain that the technology was not the therapy. The technology was a medium for a range of types of art therapy and it did not predetermine the kind of therapy that would be done with it. The research cited above, showing only small differences in relationship formation and therapeutic outcomes between different modes of mediated communication, helped shift the focus toward human factors and away from technological factors.

A Preferred Mode of Mediated Communication

It became clear that therapeutic procedures and ethical protocols would be the foundation of online art therapy rather than specific technologies. This opened the way for thinking that the best approach to online art therapy would be to use whatever communication technology is most readily available and familiar to the clients, whether this is something high-tech on a computer, phone, or other advanced device, or something low-tech using a fax machine or even paper mail.

In the world of business, a preferred mode of mediated communication took hold in those early days that reflected the research about mediated communication and provided a useful model for online art therapy. This preferred mode uses initial video contact to let people become familiar with one another and establish a level of trust, followed by voice communication without video while looking at a shared whiteboard or other shared visual. For online art therapy, this would translate to interaction with videoconferencing at the beginning, followed by voice communication without video while clients create art, and then videoconferencing again as the clients share their mark making with the therapist and other group members. In situations where videoconferencing is not possible, clients and therapists can decide whether or not to share photographs of themselves instead of having initial videoconferencing contact. Only a small amount of visual information is necessary for people to size each other up (we do this whether we intend to or not) and start building trust. It is possible to capitalize on potential advantages of no-sight communication to reduce feelings of vulnerability and promote self-disclosure, and to increase 'task focus' by reducing distractions.

Art Therapy: A Good Fit for Telehealth

The seeds of online art therapy were planted when art therapists and others embraced the possibilities of low-bandwidth forms of telehealth, such as email communication. They noticed that art therapy was a good fit for the telehealth technology of the time because of the presence of visual images. Art images could provide abundant non-verbal information and activate the sense of sight while communicating without seeing the other person or people. Art therapy is conducted in relation to images made by clients as well as in relation to art therapists. Images can easily be sent from one location to another and can be discussed and viewed simultaneously by people in different locations.

Developing Synchronous Distance Art Therapy

In 1997, Davor Čubranić and I took the opportunity to develop internet art therapy, and by 1998, we set about creating a computer program and clinical procedures for hosting synchronous art therapy groups using computers and the internet. This was an unusual interdisciplinary collaborative project between a graduate student in computer science with a specialty in human-computer interaction (Davor) and a graduate student in counselling psychology with a specialty in art therapy (me). With many test sessions along the way to de-bug the software and get feedback about how it felt to use it, we created a system for group art therapy sessions for people who were all in different locations. We called it *distance art therapy*, rather than *virtual art therapy*, because at the time, the word 'virtual' was associated mainly with virtual reality, where an artificial experience stands in for a real experience.

As far as we know, we were the first to create a way to offer online art therapy that was synchronous, in real time, rather than asynchronous with email, and the first to develop tools and procedures for online art therapy with groups. We did this within the constraints of very low bandwidth by using a simple art-making program combined with voice communication. Group members couldn't see each other, but they could speak with each other and the art therapist, and they could make art on their computers and share it with the group for discussion. It was too early to use our methods in the real world so everything we did was in interconnected computer labs.

We simultaneously developed computer technology and clinical procedures for using the technology. The art-making software was adapted from open-source paint software with tools similar to art materials that an art therapist at the time might use for group art therapy. Our goals were modest. We wanted to compare group art therapy on the internet with in-person group art therapy, so we mimicked a common style of in-person group art therapy as closely as possible. More than anything, we needed to know if online art therapy was possible. We kept the technology simple so clients and therapists would not be distracted by figuring out the technical side.

A Technical Innovation Allows a Therapeutic Innovation

Our simple paint program was coupled with voice software so anyone could speak and be heard by the others at any time. Although the art therapist could not see the people in the group, the therapist could watch the computer drawings as they were being made. This was significant from an art therapy point of view. Art therapists would not be able to witness clients' body language or facial expressions as they painted on their computers, but they could see the paintings evolve as they were being made. It was not feasible to send entire digital paintings from computer to computer during a session as it is now. Instead, what was sent from computer to computer was individual mouse movements. This technological solution to bandwidth constraints allowed the important clinical innovation of therapists being able to witness paintings being made. The art therapist could watch any painting being made at any time by clicking on an icon and opening it into a window, perhaps tiling it with other paintings.

As each person painted, the mouse movements that created a painting went to that person's computer monitor and also to the computers of the therapist and everyone else in the group. This made it possible for paintings to be passed from one group member to another for 'pass-the-painting' activities and collaborative art making. We wanted group members to be able to interact with each other in a variety of ways for group cohesion and bonding between group members. With the exception of these activities, group members wouldn't see the paintings of others until it was time to discuss them. They could see icons that let them know that other paintings were happening, a mimicking of in-person groups where members are aware that others are making art without watching what they are doing.

Input From Volunteers and Research Participants

Most of the volunteers who came to the computer lab to test the system were interdisciplinary graduate students at the University of British Columbia whose areas of study spanned two or more academic disciplines. We valued their multiple viewpoints and took to heart their reactions and spontaneous comments. Most had never used computer art software before. Several surprised us by remarking that making art with a computer gave them more access to their subconscious minds. A few said they felt less self-conscious

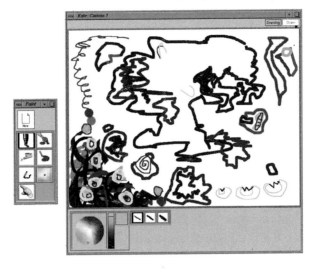

Figure 2.1 Distance Art Therapy in 1998—Author's User Interface with Her Squiggle
Drawing

making art with a computer than with regular art materials because they didn't
expect to be good at computer art. On the other hand, one said that looking at
a screen suppressed her visual imagination and told us that there had been
research showing that this can happen.

When we were ready for mock group art therapy sessions, we invited ten
research participants to role-play group art therapy clients and then discuss this
experience in focus groups. The ten people were counsellors, art therapists, and
educators, each with specific professional and/or personal experience relevant to
online art therapy for people experiencing isolation that might have been due to
illness or disability.

Focus Group Findings

The research participants identified potential problems, but quickly proposed
human solutions for most of the problems they identified. For example, when
they discussed the problem of the vulnerability a client might feel from not
knowing whether others are looking at their painting or how they are reacting,
they suggested ways to indicate when others are looking and which part of the
painting they are looking at. From this we developed procedures for "active
looking": using the pointing tool to show that you are looking at an image and to
track your gaze, and to point to the parts you are talking about when discussing
an image.

Two of our research participants were counsellors who used wheelchairs.
They saw great potential for people with disabilities who might have difficulty
leaving their homes and who might benefit from using computers for art

therapy because of the adaptive tools that exist to help people with disabilities use computers. One of them noticed how good it felt to be able to draw a perfect circle as a person with limited use of their hands.

For the ever-present problem of technical failure, research participants suggested three things: a) rehearse with each client ahead of time what to do in the event of technical failure (and use this discussion as a foundation for group building); b) have an alternate way to contact each client; and c) have the name and contact information for someone the client could turn to if they got cut off or needed assistance.

One problem that didn't have an easy solution then—and still does not—is the lack of shared physical presence. The participants in our study suggested a partial solution to this problem, which is to have people describe their surroundings. We found that this made a bigger difference than might be expected for helping people feel physically close when they don't see each other, or to bring a feeling of proximity into the therapeutic interaction. That a little thing could make such a big difference is another example of how people use what they have to steer distance communication toward uncertainty reduction, emotional closeness, and relationship formation. Nowadays, with videoconferencing, an equivalent to this might be to have people describe what is going on in their setting.

Another problem without an obvious solution had to do with technical support and confidentiality. Even today with a higher overall level of computer literacy, an online art therapy client might need technical support. If the technical support comes from someone other than the art therapist or a group member, it can be hard to protect clients' confidentiality. This puts pressure on the art therapist to acquire enough technical expertise to provide technical support while protecting confidentiality.

The Answer is Yes

By the end of our study we had an answer to our question: yes, online art therapy was possible, and it appeared to have great potential as a form of telehealth for people who would not otherwise have access to art therapy and as a type of low-bandwidth tele-therapy with a visual dimension. There was interest in commercializing our software setup, but we had learned that it was not the software that needed to be carried forward—it was the clinical procedures we had honed and the insights we had gained from our focus groups. I have done my best to present the most important of those insights here. For complete descriptions of the work that Davor and I did together and the results of the focus group studies, you can read Collie et al. (2000), which describes our project and research findings for a counselling audience, or Collie & Čubranić (1999) which was written for an art therapy audience. We also wrote about the project from a computer science perspective (Collie et al., 1998) and from a social work perspective (Collie & Čubranić, 2002).

Conclusion

This chapter and this book provide a snapshot of the development and the past and current practical and ethical considerations around delivering art therapy online to various populations. While online art therapy widens the reach of therapeutic interventions into remote communities and is able to engage clients for whom it is more difficult to attend in-person sessions, technological bottlenecks, such as connection bandwidth, and necessary know-how for client and therapist provide new challenges. Some people do not have access to the technology required or do not have a suitable private place for art therapy via videoconferencing—a problem addressed in later chapters of this book, and by Zubala and Hackett (2020)—so lower-tech alternatives need to be kept in mind. There also are situations where it is not possible or not permissible for art therapists to see their clients, or it might be possible, but not ideal. For someone whose appearance has recently changed, perhaps because of cancer treatment, or for people who have histories of being negatively judged for their appearance, no-sight communication during art therapy might have benefits. Online art therapy does not try to replace in-person art therapy sessions, but it provides another avenue of offering psychotherapy as part of a broader range of services to clients.

References

Ball, C. J., McLaren, P. M., Summerfield, A. B., Lipsedge, M. S., & Watson, J. P. (1995). A comparison of communication modes in adult psychiatry. *Journal of Telemedicine and Telecare, 1,* 22–26.

Bloom, J. W. (1998) The ethical practice of web counseling. *British Journal of Guidance & Counselling, 26*(1), 53–59.

Cervinkas, J. (1984). *Telehealth: Telecommunications technology in health care and health education in Canada.* Canadian Commission for UNESCO.

Citera, M. (1998). Distributed teamwork: The impact of communication media on influence and decision quality. *Journal of the American Society for Information Science, 49*(9), 792–800.

Cohen, G. E., & Kerr, B. A. (1998). Computer-mediated counseling: An empirical study of a new mental health treatment. *Computers in Human Services, 15*(4), 13–26.

Collie, K. (2004). Interpersonal communication in behavioral telehealth: What can we learn from other fields? In J. Bloom & G. Walz (Eds.), *Cybercounseling and Cyberlearning: An Encore* (pp. 345–365). Greensboro NC: CAPS Press and American Counseling Association.

Collie, K., & Čubranić, D. (1999). An art therapy solution to a telehealth problem. *Art Therapy: The Journal of the American Art Therapy Association, 16*(4), 186–193.

Collie, K., & Čubranić, D. (2002). Computer-supported distance art therapy: A focus on traumatic illness. *Journal of Technology in Human Services, 20*(1), 155–171.

Collie, K., Čubranić, D., & Booth, K. (1998). Participatory design of a system for computer-supported distance art therapy. In *Proceedings of the Participatory Design Conference 1998* (pp. 29–36). Seattle, WA: Computer Professionals for Social Responsibility.

Collie, K., Mitchell, D., & Murphy, L. (2000). Skills for cybercounseling: Maximum impact at minimum bandwidth. In J. Bloom & G. Walz (Eds.) *CyberCounseling and Cyberlearning: Strategies and Resources for the Millennium* (pp. 219–236). Greensboro NC: CAPS Press and American Counseling Association.

Colòn, Y. (1999). Digital digging: Group therapy online. In J. Fink (Ed.) *How to use computers and cyberspace in clinical practice of psychotherapy* (pp. 66–81). Northvale, NJ: Jason Aronson.

Day, S. X., & Schneider, P. L. (2000). The subjective experiences of therapists in face-to-face, video, and audio sessions. In J. W. Bloom & G. R. Walz (Eds.), *Cybercounseling and Cyberlearning: Strategies and Resources for the Millennium* (pp. 203–218). Greensboro NC: CAPS Press and American Counseling Association.

Doherty-Sneddon, G., Anderson, A., O'Malley, C., Langton, S., Garrod, S., & Bruce, V. (1997). Face-to-face and video-mediated communication: A comparison of dialogue structure and task performance. *Journal of Experimental Psychology: Applied*, *3*(2), 105–125.

Fish, S. L. (1990). Therapeutic uses of the telephone: Crisis intervention vs. traditional therapy. In G. Gumpert & S. L. Fish (Eds.), *Talking to Strangers: Mediated Therapeutic Communication* (pp. 154–169). Norwood, NJ: Ablex.

Graetz, K. A., Boyle, E. S., Kimble, C. E., Thompson, P., & Garloch, J. L. (1998). Information sharing in face-to-face, teleconferencing, and electronic chat groups. *Small Group Research*, *29*(6), 714–743.

Murphy, L. J., & Mitchell, D. L. (1998). When writing helps to heal: E-mail as therapy. *British Journal of Guidance and Counselling*, *26*(1), 21–32.

Robertson, T. (1997). "And it's a generalization. But no it's not:" Women, communication work and the discourses of technology design. In A. F. Grundy, D. Kohler, V. Oechtering & U. Petersen (Eds.), *Women, Work and Computerization. Proceedings of the 6th International IFIP-Conference, Bonn, Germany, May 24–27, 1997* (pp. 263–275). Berlin: Springer.

Sampson, J. P., Kolodinsky, R. W., & Greeno, B. P. (1997). Counseling and the information highway: Future possibilities and potential problems. *Journal of Counseling & Development*, *75*(3), 203–212.

Shah, S. (2016, May 14). The history of social networking. *Digital Trends*. https://www.digitaltrends.com/features/the-history-of-social-networking/.

Sproull, L., & Kiesler, S. (1996, September). Computers, networks, and work. *Scientific American*, 755–761.

Stamm, B. (1998). Clinical applications of telehealth in mental health care. *Professional Psychology: Research and Practice*, *29*, 536–542.

Walther, J. B. (1992). Interpersonal effects in computer-mediated interaction: A relational perspective. *Communication Research*, *19*(1), 52–90.

Walther, J. B. (1996). Computer-mediated communication: Impersonal, interpersonal, and hyperpersonal interaction. *Communication Research*, *23*(1), 3–43.

Walther, J. B., Anderson, J. F., & Park, D. W. (1994). Interpersonal effects in computer mediated interaction: A meta-analysis of social and antisocial communication. *Communication Research*, *21*, 460–487.

Weinberg, N. (1996). Compassion by computers: Contrasting the supportiveness of computer-mediated and face-to-face interactions. *Computers in Human Services*, *13*(2), 51–63.

Yellowlees, P., & Kennedy, C. (1996). Telemedicine applications in an integrated mental health service based at a teaching hospital. *Journal of Telemedicine and Telecare*, *2*, 205–209.

Zhu, S., Tedeschi, G., Anderson, C., & Pierce, J. (1996). Telephone counseling for smoking cessation: What's in a call? *Journal of Counseling and Development, 75*, 93–102.

Zubala, A., & Hackett, S. (2020) Online art therapy practice and client safety: A UK-wide survey in times of COVID-19. *International Journal of Art Therapy, 25*(4), 161–171, doi:10.1080/17454832.2020.1845221.

3 Online Art Therapy

Experiences of Art Therapists During the COVID-19 Pandemic

Jessica A. Walters

Introduction

This chapter offers suggestions and raises ethical considerations for a tele art therapy practice. Online approaches to art therapy are novel and I use the terms virtual, online, and tele art therapy interchangeably in this chapter. Tele art therapy, a subset of teletherapy, emerged in the late 1990s (McNiff, 1999). The bulk of art therapy literature written before the COVID-19 pandemic focuses on implementing online computer programs that can be used to facilitate art therapy and adapting analogue art therapy practices to suit online platforms. In contrast, tele art therapy literature published during the pandemic includes surveys and descriptions of art therapy programs and services developed in response to stay-at-home orders. The analysis of my research's results suggest that by conducting teletherapy, art therapists are re-conceptualizing ideas around therapeutic space, accessibility, materials, and client–therapist power dynamics. To conclude, I offer suggestions and raise ethical considerations for online art therapy practice.

Tele Art Therapy Literature Review

Kate Collie was one of the first to advocate for the use of online art therapy within the field of teletherapy in 1999 (Collie & Čubranić, 1999; Collie et al., 2007). Collie and Čubranić (1999) describe an action research study in which the authors designed and evaluated an interactive online drawing program designed for tele art therapy. Themes of "ease-of-use and lack of inhibition, social protocols, protection against misrepresentation, qualities of computer images in relation to art therapy, and feelings of mastery and control" (Collie & Čubranić, 1999, p. 190) developed from focus-group discussions. The authors argue that art therapy is "uniquely suited to Telehealth" (Collie & Čubranić, 1999, p. 191).

In 2009, Chilton et al. published an article about their involvement in an international virtual community arts studio. Through the online group, members share art project ideas and take part in exchanges where participants mail each

DOI: 10.4324/9781003149538-4

other gifts or create collaborative artworks that circulate by mail. The authors claim that through online community arts studios, "art therapists have become architects of the techno-digital culture, building online communities that encourage creativity and happiness" (Chilton et al., 2009, p. 71).

Levy et al. (2017) describe ways creative arts therapists can practice online. The authors mention a group of rural veterans who receive services from an art therapist via videoconference. All clients receive various art supplies by mail. In sessions, group participants are given art directives and are encouraged to share their completed work with the group. During discussion, the therapist shares screenshots of art images and asks the participant to describe what they see. This practice establishes "a common vocabulary and [improves] the level of communication between the therapist and the telehealth participant" (Levy et al., 2017, pp. 23–24).

In May 2020, Choudhry and Keane conducted a survey of 623 American art therapists to better understand COVID-19's impact on the art therapy profession. Results revealed that the majority of art therapists (73.2%) transitioned from in-person therapy to teletherapy during the pandemic. According to the survey, 79.8% of art therapists had difficulty viewing clients' art-making process and 78.2% of art therapists experienced challenges effectively incorporating art materials into sessions. Despite the difficulties, teletherapy has increased access to care for some clients; over one-third (37.4%) of art therapists reported that teletherapy has enabled them to offer services to clients who did not previously have access (Choudhry & Keane, 2020, p. 8).

On the other side of the Atlantic, Zubala and Hackett (2020) surveyed 96 art therapists in the United Kingdom to determine how art therapists adapted to providing online art therapy services. Survey outcomes highlighted the importance of managing online safety risks, establishing digital boundaries, and developing privacy protocols unique to online art therapy (Zubala & Hackett, 2020).

British art therapists Datlen and Pandolfi (2020) describe making online platforms more accessible to people with learning disabilities at risk for social isolation. Formed in response to social distancing orders, the studio-based art therapy group took place on the smartphone application WhatsApp. According to the authors, individuals with learning disabilities may often feel excluded from digital spaces, and the facilitated WhatsApp group allowed participants to connect with one another and share images of artwork and the adversities of COVID-19 alongside other losses (Datlen & Pandolfi, 2020).

Although limited, tele art therapy literature provides some insight into how art therapists practice online therapy. My study seeks to add to this body of research.

Methodology

Study Design

I derived my qualitative methodology from Charmaz' (2014) constructivist grounded theory. Grounded theory involves strategies of simultaneous data collection and analysis, forming codes and categories directly from the data, using comparisons during each stage of the analysis, and self-reflexive memo-writing (Charmaz, 2014). This framework is helpful where there is limited existing theory (Birks & Mills, 2015; Charmaz, 2014), and it is appropriate for my research because online art therapy is a developing field. Rather than claiming to capture an "objective" view of reality, my research focuses on the opinions and experiences of the participants.

Participants and Procedure

My sampling was purposive. Research participants were professional, American art therapists who have conducted online art therapy services during the COVID-19 pandemic. I interviewed five participants who worked in various settings with different populations. Employing the snowball sampling method, I recruited one art therapist who specialized in virtual group therapy, one who worked with families, two who worked with individuals, and one who worked in community arts. These four, broad categories represent common contexts in which professional art therapists practice.

I conducted and recorded the interviews via Google Meet, a free, video conferencing platform approved by the US Health Insurance Portability and Accountability Act (HIPAA). I downloaded a Google Meet extension that transcribed discussions in real time.

From January 2020 to March 2021, I facilitated semi structured interviews that utilized open-ended questions. All participants received the interview questions and an informed consent form that detailed the risks and benefits of participating in the research. During interviews, I asked follow-up questions and encouraged participants to elaborate on topics that felt important to them; conversations about online art therapy developed organically. I reviewed each recording and edited the transcripts for accuracy. Lastly, I emailed interview participants their transcripts to inspect.

Results

Data analysis resulted in the construction of six major themes (bolded in text):

1   Platforms
2   Navigating the virtual therapeutic space
3   Accessibility and/or inaccessibility of online art therapy
4   Coping with teletherapy challenges unique to the art therapy profession

5   Reconceptualizing materials
6   Client-therapist power differentials and cultural competence

Each theme and their subcategories aid in answering the research questions: How are art therapists in America adapting their practices as a result of the COVID-19 stay-at-home orders? How can art therapists provide telehealth services in the near future?

Research participants worked in a variety of online settings with various populations (Table 3.1). All interviewees stated that they offered art therapy services via videoconference for the first time in March or April of 2020. In addition to questions about workplaces, professional credentials, and clients, I asked participants about their self-identified gender, race, sexual orientation, and (dis)ability status (Table 3.1). These questions encouraged participants to reflect on how their intersectional identities might inform or affect their tele art therapy practices.

Art therapists described videoconferencing software as the most common **platform** used for online art therapy. In addition, the data revealed that social media were used for youth engagement. Participant 1, an art therapist who worked for a community organization that served Black and Latina girls, believes that social media is "a refreshing way to think about client engagement." Participant 1 described a private Facebook group where youth from her organization "could interact with therapeutic material," such as walking meditations, art therapy directives, and cooking videos.

The theme of **navigating the virtual therapeutic space** refers to key differences between conducting therapy online versus in person. Some art therapists reported that it was easier to solidify rapport online, while others found building rapport more difficult. Art therapists identified clients' comfortability at home and shared vulnerability as factors that cultivated the therapeutic relationship. When speaking about the benefits of online art therapy, Participant 4 stated that,

> [It's] how vulnerable it is to be right now. I'm on my couch at home doing therapy with my client, and the client is in their home. There's a sense of connection because we're all experiencing this collective trauma together.

Participant 4 sees the COVID-19 pandemic as a shared experience of trauma that enables her to relate to her clients. She notes however, that "rapport is taking longer to build [online]" than it may have in person.

Participant 5, a director of a community arts studio, expressed that conducting services online makes her feel disconnected from her participants. Throughout the interview, Participant 5 disclosed that she misses the communal experience of making art alongside regular members. She views not being able to see participants as a barrier to communication which negatively impacts rapport.

Table 3.1 Participants' Demographics and Work Setting

	Gender Identity	Race	Sexual Orientation	(Dis) ability	Other Identities	Professional License(s)	Primary Clientele	Work Setting	Therapy Focus
Participant 1	Woman	Black American	Heterosexual	No	N/A	ATR, LPC	**Current position:** adults with severe mental illnesses **Previous position:** Black and Latina youth	Partial Hospitalization, Intensive Outpatient	Groups
Participant 2	Non-binary	White	Queer	Yes	N/A	ATR, LCMHC	Queer identifying adolescents and young adults	Private Practice	Individuals
Participant 3	Woman	White	Bisexual	No	In Addiction Recovery	ATR-BC, LCPC, CADC	Low-income families and youth	Community Mental Health	Families, individuals
Participant 4	Woman	White	Heterosexual	No	Latina	N/A	Adolescent and adult survivors of sexual violence	Community Mental Health	Individuals, groups
Participant 5	Woman	White	Heterosexual	No	N/A	ATR-BC	Various	Community Arts	Groups, community arts

Four out of five art therapists mentioned maintaining confidentiality as a challenge. According to interviewees, confidentiality issues often occur because clients may not have a private space for therapy in their homes, which might lead to self-censorship, where they become less willing to disclose information for fear that someone in their home might overhear them. Some research participants navigated confidentiality issues by discussing the importance of privacy with clients' families.

Four out of five research participants had established protocols for mental health emergencies that may arise. Common protocols include verifying the client's location at the beginning of the sessions, encouraging the client to stay on screen until their emergency contact is reached, referring to the client's safety plan, and connecting the client to local emergency services.

The data reveals that tele art therapy is more **accessible** to some clients and **inaccessible** to others. Art therapists mentioned COVID safety and the ability to provide art therapy across physical distance as the most common reasons why providing online art therapy makes services more accessible. Contrarily, some participants explained how online art therapy may be inaccessible to specific clients citing financial and technological barriers and experiencing symptomatology exacerbated by technology.

From Participant 1's perspective, her workplace's virtual partial hospitalization program is growing because patients are required to attend therapy five days a week and "don't feel comfortable with COVID," despite social distancing and cleaning procedures. Furthermore, Participant 4 mentioned that offering tele art therapy services eliminated the time and money that clients would be required to spend commuting to an agency, which resulted in some clients missing fewer sessions. In contrast, Participant 5 recognized a drastic change in her clientele which reflected participants "not having access to technology" or lacking sufficient knowledge about video software to participate.

While art therapists have experienced many of the teletherapy struggles that other clinicians face, conducting virtual art therapy has forced art therapists to cope with teletherapy challenges unique to the profession, such as clients not wanting to make art in sessions. Three out of the five interviewees reported feeling underprepared to transition to distance art therapy in 2020.

With clients having limited access to art materials compared to in-person sessions, art therapists invented creative solutions by **reconceptualizing materials**. In addition to accessible and familiar materials, art therapists report clients using materials typically not associated with traditional art therapy, expanding preconceived ideas of what constitutes art materials. Other research participants have overcome this obstacle by sending art materials to clients.

Accessible and familiar materials are inexpensive materials typically found in clients' homes. Participants reported using materials in sessions that clients naturally gravitated towards, even if it meant delving into other expressive art forms beyond the visual arts. Participant 2 stated, "I've had people do cosplay makeup during sessions. I also have folks who play music, sing, or dance." Other unconventional art materials that participants used include plants, journals, and found objects.

Art therapists identified how power and cultural differences manifest within the virtual environment. Participant 2 believes "that [therapists] sit in the [virtual therapy space] with our whole selves, with all of our identities, and power and privilege come up in therapy spaces just like they do everywhere." Participant 5 expressed that the transition to online programing has made adhering to her community art studio's mission to cultivate an inclusive community more challenging. One of the main ideas of [her nonprofit] is that everyone at the studio is considered "participants," rather than studio leaders and customers. She expressed that when offering virtual arts programing, if there are "no designated leaders, it's really kind of bizarre, so [my colleagues and I] have really had to say that we are facilitators."

When asked how art therapists might provide culturally relevant services to their clients via teletherapy platforms, four out of five interviewees recommended allowing clients time in sessions to address culturally relevant issues. Culturally relevant issues that interviewees mentioned include cultural events, cultural holidays, family and family obligations, political movements, topics in the news, and discussing what *home* means to clients.

The six overarching themes that emerged from the data provide valuable insights into how art therapists have adapted their practices to suit online formats during the COVID-19 pandemic, which will be further discussed in the next section.

Discussion

My research participants explained that offering tele art therapy has increased access to mental healthcare to some clients, while their clients' financial struggles or symptomatology makes teletherapy inaccessible to others. These findings correspond with Choudhry and Keane's (2020) American Art Therapy Association survey. Interestingly, my research respondents stated that their clients' lack of access to tele art therapy relates to clients' marginalized identities, notably, low socioeconomic status (SES) or specific physical disabilities. This information corresponds to Usiskin and Lloyd's (2020) claim that providing online art therapy has revealed notable social inequalities regarding technology access.

Regarding community arts, creating an inclusive community might be challenging to achieve through virtual programing. First of all, low SES participants may lack the technology to engage in virtual programing. Second, according to Participant 5, the nature of video conferencing requires a clear, primary facilitator; working on artwork in a collaborative and nonhierarchical way might be difficult in this context. Thus, interviewees' comments about client–therapist power dynamics conflict with the idea of Chilton et al. (2009) that online spaces are more "egalitarian" (p. 66).

There are two notable weaknesses of my study. First, the sample size of five is not large enough to make sweeping claims about American art therapists practicing online art therapy. Secondly, my personal experiences as a teletherapy client have caused me to view it favourably. By engaging in self-reflexive memo writing and coding close to the data, I have attempted to minimize my biases.

Recommendations

Before starting a virtual art therapy session, I recommend that clinicians confirm their client's location and ask the client if they are in a private space. Should a household member in the client's or therapist's home be able to overhear the session, art therapists should wear headphones and encourage the client to do the same. Before beginning tele art therapy with a new client, art therapists must clearly articulate the limits of online confidentiality within the consent for treatment form. Art therapists may also verbally explain the importance of privacy during therapy to clients and their household members.

Art therapists must have protocols for emergency situations that may arise during online sessions. In addition to verifying the location of the client, other possible safety protocols include encouraging the client to stay on screen until their emergency contact is reached, referring to the client's safety plan (if applicable), and connecting the client to local emergency services. Art therapists practicing virtually may live far away from their clients; for this reason, art therapists should familiarize themselves with emergency resources and referrals in their clients' vicinity.

Art therapists should expect that each client may respond to tele art therapy differently. Rapport might be easier to build with some clients and take more time to build with others via teletherapy. I suggest that art therapists check in regularly with clients regarding how they feel about tele art therapy and the status of the therapeutic relationship.

To strengthen rapport and avoid causing harm to clients, art therapists should allow clients to process culturally relevant material in virtual sessions. This includes discussing significant cultural holidays, political events, and encounters with racism, sexism, ableism, or other oppressive structures. Encounters with oppressive structures happen outside as well as within the virtual therapeutic space.

Regarding materials, clients may make art over videoconferences, share artwork via secure texting platforms, or describe their artwork over the phone. If clients lack art supplies, art therapists may advocate for agency funding to mail clients materials. Additionally, art therapists may encourage clients to use forms of creative expression that clients find familiar and accessible. An example that research participants gave for software that can be used to create digital artwork is Jamboard, a free, interactive whiteboard by Google Suite. Jamboard allows art therapists and clients to draw on a digital page simultaneously. Art therapists can also use free smartphone applications or utilize other social media platforms as appropriate.

Furthermore, if art therapists encourage clients to use art making as a coping skill, art therapists should support clients in honing artistic skills with materials that they have easy access to outside of therapy. This way, clients can readily *apply* the coping skill that they have learned in art therapy on their own.

Conclusion

The lack of literature on online art therapy and research participants' remarks about feeling underprepared to transition to teletherapy underscores that more research must be conducted on the subject. Going forward, graduate-level coursework in the field should address virtual art therapy and training on how to conduct art therapy online should be implemented. Other opportunities to learn about virtual therapy may include consulting with other clinicians and completing online training programs for tele counselling.

This research will benefit art therapists and their clients by extension. The analysis reflects that art therapists who have facilitated online art therapy during the pandemic have adapted their practices by thinking about accessibility, materials, and client-therapist power dynamics in new ways. After the COVID-19 pandemic ends and people may return to some semblance of normal life, art therapists who have experience conducting art therapy online will be able to serve clients that they have not served before. Art therapists must cater their practices to meet the current needs of their clients. This research gives art therapists some guidance on how to adapt their practices to suit online formats, so that they can best meet their clients' needs in these changing times.

References

Birks, M., & Mills, J. (2015). *Grounded theory: A practical guide*. Sage Publications.

Charmaz, K. (2014). *Constructing grounded theory: A practical guide through qualitative analysis*. Sage Publications.

Chilton, G., Gerity, L., LaVorgna-Smith, M., & MacMichael, H. (2009). An online art exchange group: 14 secrets for a happy artist's life. *Art Therapy: Journal of the American Art Therapy Association, 26*(2), 66–72. https://doi.org/10.1080/07421656.2009.10129741

Choudhry, R., & Keane, C. (2020). *Art therapy during a mental health crisis: Coronavirus pandemic impact report*. The American Art Therapy Association. https://arttherapy.org/upload/Art-Therapy-Coronavirus-Impact-Report.pdf.

Collie, K., & Čubranić, D. (1999) An art therapy solution to a telehealth problem, *Art Therapy: Journal of the American Art Therapy Association, 16*(4) 186–193, https://doi.org/10.1080/07421656.1999.10129481.

Collie, K., Kreshka, M., Ferrier, S., Parsons, R., Graddy, K., Avram, S., Mannell, P., Chen, X., Perkins, J., & Koopman, C. (2007). Videoconferencing for delivery of breast cancer support groups to women living in rural communities: a pilot study. *Psycho-Oncology, 16*(8), 778–782. doi:10.1002/pon.1145

Datlen, G., & Pandolfi, C. (2020). Developing an online art therapy group for learning disabled young adults using WhatsApp. *International Journal of Art Therapy, 25*(4), 192–201.

McNiff, S. (1999). The virtual art therapy studio. *American Journal of Art Therapy, 16*(4), 197–200.

Levy, C., Spooner, H., Lee, J., Sonke, J., Myers, K., & Snow, E. (2017). Telehealth-based creative arts therapy: Transforming mental health and rehabilitation care for rural veterans. *The Arts in Psychotherapy, 57*, 20–26. doi:10.1016/j.aip.2017.08.010.

Usiskin, M., & Lloyd, B. (2020). Lifeline, frontline, online: Adapting art therapy for social engagement across borders. *International Journal of Art Therapy*, *25*(4), 183–191. https://doi.org/10.1080/17454832.2020.1845219.

Zubala, A., & Hackett, S. (2020). Online art therapy practice and client safety: a UK-wide survey in times of COVID-19. *International Journal of Art Therapy*, *25*(4), 161–171. https://doi.org/10.1080/17454832.2020.1845221.

Section 2

Clinical Perspectives

4 Borders and Boundaries in Virtual Art Therapy

With excerpts of an interview with Girija Kaimal conducted in November 2020

Michelle Winkel

Introduction

Most of the authors in this book and many of our readers are seasoned art therapists, long familiar with the art table at which we sit with our clients, covered in art materials that we can touch, smell, and lovingly present to our clients in our face-to-face studios. The pandemic has thrust upon us the requirement to practice differently and this change challenges us in many ways.

Virtual art therapy has seemingly deconstructed borders everywhere, promising to reach those previously unable to obtain services, whether due to barriers, such as stigma or inability to travel, or those who are isolated because of their physical disability, age, or illness (Peterson, 2010, p. 28; Kaimal et al., 2019, p. 19). All that is required is an adequate internet connection and a computer or mobile device. This gives art therapists more potential to serve clients outside of their geographical area, and therefore increases the likelihood that therapists are ethnically, culturally, religiously, and/or socio-economically different from their clients. Furthermore, virtual art therapy, because of its increasing worldwide access, is uniquely positioned to reach clients who might otherwise not seek art therapy. It can be provided at extremely low costs as technology advances, giving access to more people.

The ability to span physical distance means we are instantly brought into much more intimate conversations with diverse clients with different cultures and languages than we have in the past. This challenges us in exciting and unpredictable ways. Reflections on this shift, and the implications of virtual practice on our prior concepts of borders and boundaries in our work, became the focus of my interview with Dr. Girija Kaimal in November 2020. Kaimal is a leading researcher, and the Assistant Dean for Special Research Initiatives, Creative Arts Therapy graduate program at Drexel University in Philadelphia.

This interview, research from The Proulx Foundation's Virtual Art Therapy Clinic (VATC), case vignettes, as well as references from current literature inform this chapter. I will focus on the concepts of cultural competence and cultural humility, which help art therapists navigate the increasingly diverse cultural landscapes of the client–art therapist relationship in the new global world of virtual art therapy. I will also argue that art making and creativity, the

DOI: 10.4324/9781003149538-6

core of our work as art therapists, is a key resource to help us navigate these cultural divisions and build relationships in a therapeutic context that spans boundaries and crosses borders. The practice of making art compliments the curiosity, openness, and exploration valued in these concepts of cultural humility and competence in a way that spoken language alone does not.

Other unique features of working via videoconference that I will discuss in this chapter are:

1   The value of expanding our assumptions of media and materials beyond western traditions
2   Issues of space, place, and language
3   Themes of trust and safety
4   Shifting and reworking the personal and professional delineation in the therapeutic relationship

The following section will introduce the VATC as a means to reach art therapy clients online and discuss the clinic's approach regarding cultural competence and cultural humility.

Virtual Art Therapy Clinic

The VATC was founded in the first weeks of the COVID pandemic by the Proulx Foundation, a not-for-profit organization in British Columbia, Canada, to provide low-cost videoconference-based art therapy to clients across Canada and other countries. It serves clients in multiple languages with approximately 15 postgraduate art therapy students who are also based in several countries, such as Canada, the UK, India, Malaysia, Saudi Arabia, Egypt, Sweden, the USA and Japan. At the time of this writing, the clinic had provided services to over a hundred clients. By July 2021, 1400 sessions had been conducted in English, Hindi, French, Cantonese, Punjabi, Hindi, Mandarin, and Arabic. The VATC website is written in English, reflecting the role of English as the predominant language at the clinic. Some of the student therapists, however, provide their biographies and video introductions in their own primary languages. The Proulx Foundation has had an international focus since its inception when it founded an in-person training program in Bangkok with Dr. Patcharin Sughondhabirom, which will be discussed in a different chapter of this book. The Foundation also established another training program in Tokyo.

The broad reach that the VATC achieves means we, as art therapists, have an increased responsibility to use models, such as cultural competence and cultural humility, to inform our practice. These two theoretical models have been used in mental health, including art therapy, to guide cross-cultural practice. They enable us to acknowledge the complexities and build tools and understanding for these situations in art therapy practice.

In her book *Cultural Humility in Art Therapy: Applications for Practice, Research, Social Justice, Self-Care, and Pedagogy*, Jackson (2020) shares that both humility and competence are both needed in cultural approaches to art therapy practice. Cultural competence is commonly defined as "the acquired knowledge that people use to interpret their world and generate social behaviour" (Spradley & McCurdy, 2012, p. 9) and "a set of congruent behaviours, attitudes and policies that come together in a system, agency or among professionals that enable that system, agency or professions to work effectively in cross-cultural situations" (Cross et al., 1989, p. 13). Cultural competence, however, is described by some as too binary a construct, implying that if one is not culturally competent, they are implicitly incompetent, and perhaps not equipped to interact professionally with members of particular groups (Chavez, 2018).

Cultural humility, on the other hand, supports curiosity, openness, and exploration when working cross-culturally, with values not disparate from creativity and art making at its core. Bal and Kaur (2018) describe it as a critical reflection regarding personal and systemic biases, and a respectful approach to relationships based on mutuality that interrogates cultural assumptions and judgments. It values learning through reciprocal relationships rather than the acquisition of factual knowledge pertaining to a particular culture. The foundation of cultural humility is the awareness that we are never finished— we do not arrive at a point when our cultural education is complete (Winkel, 2018). Thus, while competence implies an arrival point in skill development, which, I believe, is impossible, cultural humility encourages a self-reflective stance of ongoing exploration. Although there is a controversy between these concepts, the VATC feels that drawing on their insights to fine-tune therapeutic practices will improve service delivery to clients.

The VATC is a training site staffed, in part, by graduate-level student art therapists. Students receive ongoing clinical supervision and have many opportunities to learn about how best to work, reflect, learn, and practice art therapy online. After each session, they complete chart notes in a secure platform used by the clinic called *Jane* (https://jane.app). They also make their own response art and upload it into each chart note. Group supervision explores the clients' art and students' response artwork together with peers and registered art therapy supervisors. Supervisors and student art therapists at the VATC are experiencing how the online delivery of art therapy brings the need for cultural humility and competence to the forefront in ways that location-based practice has generally not required.

This can include how we choose materials and media in the work of art therapy. In my interview with Kaimal, we explored the sometimes Eurocentric assumptions about media and materials. She said,

> When we show up with our structured media like pencil crayons, markers, paint—our idea of structured media is very Western. What about traditional art forms that use natural materials, like rangoli or henna in India, or wall paintings? To really recognize that art therapy was created in a Western context, and to allow for the possibility that many of the things that we hold to be true might need to be let go.

Students at the VATC are encouraged to approach all of their sessions with cultural humility *and* competence, which includes selecting art materials and activities that align with the client's situation, circumstance, finances, culture, therapeutic goals, and interests. Competence asks of the students that they have read about and studied the culture of their clients. Humility asks that they stay open and reflect on the materials that the client wants to work with, even if the student is not as comfortable or familiar with it.

Hedaya AlDaleel, a VATC therapist, wanted to practice a specific art activity she had learned in class with her 43-year-old Arab male client whom we will call Raman. She had been working with him for about five weeks online at the clinic. She realized that the activity of selecting an animal to represent each of his family members and himself might be offensive to him. In Arab culture, according to AlDaleel, identifying someone as an animal is not respectful. AlDaleel knew she couldn't approach the activity the same way she did with her Western clientele. Instead, she asked him to imagine a younger version of himself, when he was six or seven years old, playing with playdoh and creating animals that represented his family members, which was eagerly accepted. The client even added humour to the process, laughing as he imagined the reactions of his family members if they were to see the animals he created to represent them. AlDaleel utilized her familiarity and competence with her client's culture, and her own humble and exploratory attitude to adapt the activity to suit the client.

The cultural implications of spoken language also play a critical role in virtual art therapy. Probably more than in face-to-face art therapy, the therapist relies on verbal cues to understand what's happening for the client. The therapist usually cannot see the client's face and artwork at the same time, unless the client has two cameras. Asking the client to describe parts of their body that are difficult to see, such as their legs, feet, and posture, may help. AlDaleel works with clients in Arabic or in English, and occasionally both. Sometimes this shared mother-tongue facilitates a stronger therapeutic alliance, and yet also gives some of her clients a chance to distance themselves from the associations or stigma their mother tongue may hold for them. For example, she works with Egyptian clients living in Canada who prefer to speak to her in English, though they occasionally lapse into Arabic, and may use Arabic in their artwork.

> Using the English language rather than Arabic often enables the clients to create a barrier in their minds, and possibly imagine a more Westernized persona to open up and discuss issues that may be considered inappropriate or taboo if discussed in Arabic.
>
> (H. AlDaleel, personal communication, 5 May 2021)

"Research has suggested that for many individuals, taboo topics may generate less anxiety for people when discussed in a foreign language" (2015, p. 462), noted Kapasi and Melluish in a systematic review. "Oftentimes, if the clients start to use the Arabic language, they quickly switch to English, and it's almost always as they discuss something more intimate or personal" (H. AlDaleel, personal communication, 2021).

Another example of AlDaleel applying cultural humility and competence to her virtual art therapy sessions can be seen with client Assa. After atypically cancelling a couple of sessions with AlDaleel, the client disclosed that her mother-in-law was visiting and that Assa didn't have a private space to open her computer and see AlDaleel for their usual session time. The client was often repeatedly interrupted by her mother-in-law, who was curious about Assa's requests for "quiet time." After brainstorming together, it was decided that Assa would wait until her mother-in-law left in two weeks to resume sessions. The stigma of receiving mental health services was too uncomfortable for the client and not an accepted solution to mental health issues within Middle Eastern culture, according to AlDaleel (personal communication, 10 June 2021). She reports that in her experience, it is not common for clients from the Middle East to discuss their mental health with family or friends. There is often a fear of judgement. Yet, the client was able to work freely in the sessions with AlDaleel, as Figure 4.1 shows.

Another example of creatively navigating how to cross virtual borders of culture and language shows up in the following session with Martina. Martina, AlDaleel's client from Argentina, uses English in sessions; both women are fluent despite the fact that English is their second language. Occasionally, Martina says, "I must teach you Spanish, Hedaya! Then you would know the names of these birds you hear outside my window when they're singing to me." For AlDaleel, this brings a richness and enjoyment to the relationship she had not anticipated. She believes that naming and exploring their differences builds a stronger therapeutic alliance and leads to better outcomes for the client.

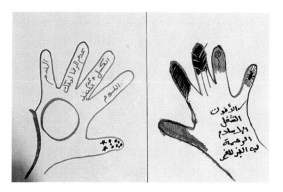

Figure 4.1 Things to Release (Left Hand) vs Things to Hold on to (Right Hand)
Note: The left hand lists the things that need to be released, including self-blame, guilt, and lack of gratitude. The right hand lists all the things the client wanted to hold on to and is grateful for, including family, inner peace, and mercy.

For some clients, naming and exploring the cultural differences in the therapeutic relationship comes naturally and easily. Ashley Nelson, a VATC art therapy student residing in Canada, was working with Saleem, a seven-year-old client in Africa in dyadic sessions with his father. One day Saleem became very interactive with Nelson during a free play session. During the play, he asked her several questions about herself. "Where do you live?" he asked her. "Is it dark outside where you are too?" and "Do you have a car?" To which Nelson replied happily, "Yes, I do have a car!"

"Only one?!" he asked mischievously.

"Yes, only one. How many do you have?" Nelson prompted.

"Three!" With his father beside him, he began to list off each cars' colour. "And one of them is white, like you!" he finished nonchalantly, turning his attention immediately back to his play.

It was interesting to observe this young client remarking on the difference in their skin tones as a matter of fact rather than a barrier between them. He also noticed the geographical distance when asking about darkness and the time of day for Nelson. He could glimpse light coming through her window and it aroused enough curiosity for him to comment. He understood she was in a very different place than he was. For other clients, obvious and subtle cultural differences are often not as comfortable to name, or even to acknowledge, whether due to racism or due to their own lived experience. Because trust and safety within the therapeutic relationship are pivotal to treatment outcomes, we want clients to feel they have choices in who they work with. A detailed biography with a photo and a video of the student therapists introducing themselves is one way to help the client get a feel for the therapist and open the door to developing a connection

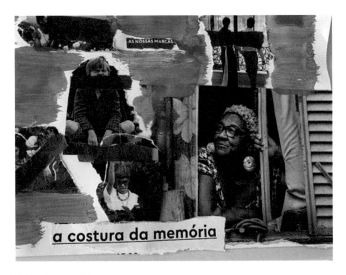

Figure 4.2 Sewing the Memories
Note: In this piece, the client used red tape to express the many times she was discouraged from using her voice.

and therapeutic alliance. The real testing ground, however, is the first session because it is not only the client who chooses the therapist, but the therapist also must feel they can work compatibly with the client.

Valerie Behiery, a French and English-speaking multi-faith woman living in Riyadh, Saudi Arabia, logs on to her VATC sessions with clients in Saudi Arabia, Egypt, India, and other countries. She works, for example, with Violet, a Saudi-raised university student in her twenties now based in Cairo. Violet received a very westernized education in Riyadh and is more fluent in English than Arabic. Violet and Behiery, as part of their sessions, have discussed the intersection of cultures that they share. This has played a critical role in the building and consolidation of a strong therapeutic relationship. At the time of this writing, Violet was studying to become a pharmacist. The fact that Violet studies a discipline more related to family expectations than to her own personal interests and inherent creative skills also constituted a rich starting point for art therapy. It provided a clear metaphor of her core challenges relating to self-identity and complex family relationships.

In virtual art therapy, Behiery introduced Violet to many traditional and non-traditional art media. Ultimately, Violet was most attracted to non-traditional materials, such as video drama-based art, and pizza dough sculptures, perhaps because they diverged from her family's more academic and traditional expectations. The video work, which the two women experimented with during online sessions, seemed to work well for Violet partly because she loves acting and storytelling. The video dramas she scripted and enacted in front of Behiery, sometimes with puppets and other props, were externalizations of her inner emotions, memories, and thoughts. The more directly accessed performative and somatic dimensions of the media seemed to help Violet explore her interests and strengths while moving toward her therapeutic goals more fully. Unlike AlDaleel's clients' use of switching from native language to second language to attain a greater sense of freedom and privacy from personal and cultural constrictions, Violet attained this freedom through her choice of diverse non-traditional media, and her therapeutic alliance with a therapist to whom she could relate.

The utilization of non-traditional media requires added faith in the creative process and in the art therapist who witnesses that process. In my interview with Kaimal, she talks about how exploration in art making can build understanding, openness, and connection, all of which are needed when working with clients of diverse cultures and backgrounds:

> What I've been trying to do is always explore art media and keep that exploratory frame in mind. Exploring media also means being open to people in all their differences and nuances. When I stay open to the art making process, I stay open to the possibilities of people.

When I asked her to expand on her role, she continued,

I think about my role mainly in the field as a researcher. I do clinical work, but it's not been my focus. I'm also an active artist, so I think that piece is really important for us as clinicians to be active in our art form. If you're not active in your art form, you don't appreciate the nuances of what art media can do for you. I see this sometimes in my students or colleagues. People have their preferred forms—which is fine, everyone has their preferred forms—and that gets thrust on patients and clients because you know that form really well and you push for that, and that may or may not be the right media.

As a clinical supervisor, I encourage my students at the VATC to explore art media through response art as a resource, to stay connected to their own feelings about clients, sort through transference and countertransference, and to build empathy and understanding. We invite the students to share their own art in supervision and other platforms in school forums, knowing it is integral to the formation of their ongoing art therapist identities.

In early studies on the strengths and challenges of teletherapy, Sampson et al. (1997) observed the reduced power imbalance between clients and therapists when compared with face-to-face sessions. Dr. Kaimal speaks about this dynamic with respect to the cultural nuances we are experiencing at the VATC, and the cautions of leaning on old theoretical traditions. She shares: "If you were taught psychodynamically, you don't reveal anything. But if you go around the world, nobody will trust you if you don't reveal anything." According to our students and researchers at VATC, there is a dropping of formality which comes with the computer screen as the portal to sitting in each other's private homes. It thereby creates a sense of experimentation with media that we feel happens more easily in virtual art therapy. For example, Behiery noticed that exploring performance-based video work with her client was much more likely through the virtual platform than it would have been face-to-face. It was possible to be transported outside of the constraints of cultural and familial norms, for a few moments, as she sat with Violet together in each session.

To emphasize the global potential of virtual art therapy, and the value of cultural humility in choosing suitable media and materials in virtual art therapy, we will discuss Behiery's client Maryam. At the time of writing this chapter, Maryam was living in India. Being the youngest child of her family, she is the only one still living with her parents. Like Violet, Maryam is a university student in a discipline chosen by her parents rather than herself, which caused much stress and difficulty. This was further complicated by a diagnosis of obsessive compulsive disorder. While she has had one session of verbal therapy outside of the home, the 24-year-old is now literally confined to her home, not due to the COVID-19 lockdowns, but because of the traditional cultural norms of her family. The COVID lockdown at the time meant that she had no access to additional art materials, except what she already had when she began art therapy, namely lined paper, coloured pencils, and tiny tubes of paint. As a result, Maryam could only obtain alternative art materials, such as recycled boxes, aluminum foil for prints or sculpting, or dry lentils for mini-installations. To accommodate the situation, Behiery introduced the digital whiteboard, photography, and the use of objects in her room like socks or scarves for art-making.

Maryam had not done art since primary school. She chose to depict stick-like figures because of her conscious and unconscious fear of her emotions stemming from ongoing trauma, as well as to Muslim aniconic religio-cultural norms regarding figurative depictions. Maryam's art and words displayed, from the first meeting, a cognizance of her inner issues due to various forms of family abuse both from parents and siblings. For example, "Wanting Mum's Love" (Figure 4.3) visually enacts her unfulfilled need for maternal love. Behiery noticed that Maryam had a gift for writing fairly early on and integrated free verse, spoken word, and haiku into the sessions in the form of graphic storytelling. In the ninth session, Behiery asked Maryam if she was open to experiencing a visualisation, and she agreed. It is a classic activity Behiery learned in class by Violet Oaklander, a European therapist and author, that guides the client to visualize and then draw a rosebush. However, Maryam raised an important cultural point during the visualization, asking if she could envision herself as a hibiscus because she had never seen a rosebush (Figure 4.4). This highlighted how Eurocentric aspects of well-known art therapy activities can be easily overlooked.

A similar situation happened with Anjanadevi Badrinath, an art therapist at the VATC working from her home in India. She had a client also situated in India and wanted to practice an art directive using plasticine, a colourful moulding material available in North America, that she had learned about in class. Her client had no access to this material, so Badrinath helped her client discover the use of chapatti dough as a substitute material similar to playdough.

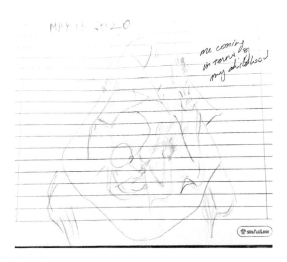

Figure 4.3 Wanting Mum's Love

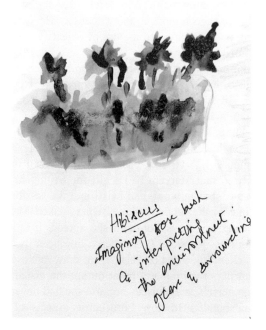

Figure 4.4 Rosebush-Hibiscus Activity

Her comfort adapting the activity to suit the client's situation built up her own confidence and fostered creative thinking in the rest of the supervision group, with whom she shared her success.

As is evident in these client vignettes, researchers AlDaleel, Nelson, Behiery, and Badrinath adopted and went beyond the concepts of cultural humility and cultural competence by maximizing their own creativity and that of their clients during each session. They kept art making central to the therapeutic process, adapted art media to both culture and circumstance, and found these choices to be ways of adapting their own worldviews to those of their clients. Using response art, supervision, and learnings from their coursework, these students became researchers in how to best deliver online art therapy to clients across the world.

Another important dynamic we notice in our clinic relates to how we contemplate and deal with 'visiting' our clients in their homes, a significant departure from face-to-face clinic-based therapy. Brandoff and Lombardi (2012) address the influence of having one's home on display through a webcam. Despite home as a familiar setting, it made Brandoff and Lombardi's research participants in the study considerably aware of the presentation of their surroundings (p. 94). This is a factor that may be disconcerting within a therapy setting, as clients have to expose their own personal space to the therapist. Yet, for clients, this may also improve aspects of safety in the therapeutic relationship. Considering the client's home environment by the therapist is referred to as an opportunity to establish deeper trust (Levy et al., 2018) and a case study of a female veteran confirmed that her progress was greatly facilitated by the opportunity to invite the art therapist into her home (Spooner et al., 2019). Clients may feel empowered by sharing more about themselves and have healing happen right where they (literally) are in their lives. Similarly, therapists may enhance the sense of trust by sharing their space with the client, which conveys aspects of their own life not typically seen in a face-to-face office visit. I encourage my students to give clients a virtual tour of their home office/studio when they start working together. Virtual touring also offers a means to establish both relational intimacy and supervisory rapport for me with my students. On the other hand, meeting in one's home office and studio, which in our case were not areas of professional domain, meant that the space had to be consciously made more appropriate for conducting art therapy and supervision.

In virtual art therapy sessions, we typically make an acknowledgement, particularly when meeting a client for the first time, about where we are, what time of day it is for us, and ask them where they're sitting. Are they in their own home or their families' home? Who is in the home at the moment? What do they see around them now—is it raining or sunny? Cold or warm? Are birds flying outside their window? For Canadians on First Nations land, we commonly make a land acknowledgement as a way to pay homage to the land, and acknowledge those who have inhabited it before Canadian settlers arrived. This act has also come to represent a way to personalize our place, as well as ground ourselves in an online environment.

Some studies found a positive impact on developing therapeutic rapport in virtual art therapy (Orr, 2012; Levy et al., 2018; Spooner et al., 2019). The use of technology in therapy was seen by some as comforting and actually helpful in reducing a client's resistance to therapy and art making (Orr, 2012). In addition to adding new demands for cross-border and cross-cultural awareness and creativity, the shift to a virtual practice of art therapy also offers an opportunity to re-examine the boundaries and norms of art therapy from its traditional Western lens.

In my interview with Kaimal, we discussed how the digital realm has moved us as therapists further into these new territories. This includes the crossing of a familiar line regarding what is "professional" in the therapeutic context. Kaimal discusses the sense of privilege she feels "to be able to talk to someone in their home and for them to talk to you in your home. That, again, breaks the therapy boundary barrier." This is counter to the traditional psychodynamic relationships in which "we only meet in the office," where "I don't know anything about your life, you don't know anything about my life." She continues, "Well, we blew that up. I'm in your home and you're in my home, and we're real people, with pets and kids and things happening in the background. What an unbreakable boundary that we broke, this idea of personal and professional. These are all good things. Why are we not accepting the extensions of our lives into our professional practice? It's not a bad thing." She continues,

It can free you from a lot of judgement. For example, all you see of me is this much. I'm sitting in my family room. My daughter is in an online school. If I were meeting you in person, I would have felt a lot more pressure to tidy up everything. Do I look okay? Am I dressed okay? A lot of those are reduced. In-person is not always the greatest, and online is not always the worst. There's so much freedom to be able to do this.

When you're online, you're also revealing aspects of your home life that you might not otherwise have. It's always telling to me when people put up that virtual background. Some things look great and some things look messy, and that's just who I am. But a lot of people spend a lot of time setting up that virtual background, and to me, that's actually telling. Why do you want to do that? Why wouldn't you want to reveal what is going on? And I have an answer to that, but it just makes me think about who works really hard to put up a virtual background and who doesn't. There's a lot we need to rethink. Approaching it with humility and recognizing that there may be many different ways that are considered professional around the world in other contexts.

Conclusion

Art therapy in virtual space offers challenges and complexities related to art media, power imbalances, space, location, language, and cultural differences, and assumptions of traditional eurocentric art therapy, to name a few. It challenges us to look at our assumptions through our own cultural lens. The power and adaptability of art making is our superpower, as evidenced by the client vignettes shared in this chapter. We can name and express the complexities inside ourselves and between each other, across borders and boundaries, and in each other's homes across the world.

In this chapter, I have shared how researchers at CiiAT's Virtual Art Therapy Clinic use cultural humility and competence, creativity, and art making as frameworks to create stronger therapeutic alliances with their diverse clients. Several themes emerged in their clinical work that were also echoed in the words of Kaimal during my interview with her. They are:

1   Using non-traditional art materials often bridge differences between client and art therapist
2   Acknowledging our place, physical space, and embracing the clients' choice of language usually deepens the therapeutic rapport
3   Staying open to possibilities through art making increases trust and safety
4   Shifting and reworking the personal and professional delineation in the therapeutic relationship has noticeable advantages and aligns with a decolonizing, culturally humble approach that we seek at the VATC

Kaimal comments on the shift in our practices from in-person to virtual due to the pandemic: "It's all uncharted territory. We're still trying to figure out the strengths and weaknesses. Online art therapy is not about being a cheaper alternative to in-person; it has unique strengths. There are things that we can do online that are very different. And what a privilege!" Therefore, art therapists, students, and clients working virtually will continue to learn about each other and themselves, and experiment together, across the globe.

References

Bal, J., & Kaur, R. (2018). Cultural humility in art therapy and child and youth care: Reflections on practice by Sikh women (L'humilité culturelle en art-thérapie et les soins aux enfants et aux jeunes: Réflexions sur la pratique de femmes sikhes). *Canadian Art Therapy Association Journal, 31*(1), 6–13. https://doi.org/10.1080/08322473.2018.1454096.

Brandoff, R., & Lombardi, R. (2012). Miles apart: Two art therapists' experience of distance supervision. *Art Therapy: Journal of the American Art Therapy Association, 29*(2), 93–96.

Chavez, V. (2018). Cultural humility: Reflections and relevance for CBPR. In N. Wallerstein, B. Duran, J. Oetzel, & M. Minkler (Eds.), *Community-based participatory research for health: Advancing social and health equity* (3rd ed., pp. 357–362). San Francisco, CA: Jossey-Bass.

Cross, T. L., Bazron, B.J., Dennis, K. W., & Isaacs, M. R. (1989). *Towards a culturally competent system of care: A monograph on effective services for minority children who are severely emotionally disturbed* (Vol. 1). Washington, DC: Georgetown University Child Development Centre.

Jackson, L. C. (2020). *Cultural humility in art therapy: Applications for practice, research, social justice, self-care, and pedagogy.* Jessica Kingsley Publishers.

Kaimal, G., Carroll-Haskins, K., Berberian, M., Dougherty, A., Carlton, N., & Ramakrishnan, A. (2020). Virtual reality in art therapy: A pilot qualitative study of the novel medium and implications for practice. *Art Therapy, 37*(1), 16–24. doi:10.1080/07421656.2019.1659662.

Kapasi, Z., & Melluish, S. (2015). Language switching by bilingual therapists and its impact on the therapeutic alliance within psychological therapy with bilingual clients: A systematic review. *International Journal of Culture and Mental Health, 8*(4), 458–477. doi:10.1080/17542863.2015.1041994.

Levy, C. E., Spooner, H., Lee, J. B., Sonke, J., Myers, K., & Snow, E. (2018). Telehealth-based creative arts therapies: Transforming mental health and rehabilitation care for rural veterans. *The Arts in Psychotherapy, 57*, 20–26. doi:10.1016/ j.aip.2017.08.010.

Orr, P. (2012). Technology use in art therapy practice: 2004 and 2011 comparisons. *The Arts in Psychotherapy, 39*(4), 234–238.

Peterson, B. C. (2010). The media adoption stage model of technology for art therapy. *Art Therapy, 27*(1), 26–31. https://doi.org/10.1080/07421656.2010.10129565.

Sampson, J. P., Kolodinsky, R. W., & Greeno, B. P. (1997). Counseling on the information highway: Future possibilities and potential problems. *Journal of Counseling & Development, 75*(3), 203–212. https://doi.org/10.1002/j.1556-6676.1997.tb02334.x.

Spooner, H., Lee, J. B., Langston, D. G., Sonke, J., Myers, K. J., & Levy, C. E. (2019). Using distance technology to deliver the creative arts therapies to veterans: Case studies in art, dance/movement and music therapy. *Arts Psychotherapy, 62*, 12–18. doi:10.1016/j.aip.2018.11.012.

Spradley, J. P., & McCurdy, D. W. (Eds.). (2012). *Conformity and conflict: Readings in cultural anthropology* (14th ed). Pearson.

Winkel, M. (2018). Musing on cultural humility (miser sur l'humilité culturelle). *Canadian Art Therapy Association Journal*, *31*(1), 1–5. doi:10.1080/08322473.2018.1458541.

5 Virtual Art Therapy with Children, Teens, and Families

A New Framework for Clinical Practice

Kathryn Snyder

Introduction

Therapists in many fields have been using telecommunication tools for some time to engage clients (Spivak et al., 2020). Art therapists, however, have not been quick to adopt teletherapy because of the use of art making and attention to sensory processes in the sessions. A lack of recent data makes it unclear how many art therapists had been utilizing telecommunication tools, such as text, audio, and video, in their practices, although a coronavirus impact report from the American Art Therapy Association (Choudry & Keane, 2021) found that many of the 623 art therapists surveyed reported transitioning to a form of teletherapy.

While acknowledging the benefit of online practices for greater access (Levy et al., 2018), there are still drawbacks to consider in the use of teletherapy, including limitations to sensing body language and expression, lack of direct eye contact with clients, difficulty managing crisis situations, and privacy/confidentiality issues. For art therapists, there are additional challenges around the use of materials and media. With children, the concern for their need for movement and play, attention spans, screen time, and ability to navigate a digital platform make virtual therapy even more challenging.

Theoretical Framework of Child/Teen and Family Art Therapy

Work with children means attention to the relational (Gerlitz et al., 2020; Ray, 2018) and ecological (Boszmorenyi-Nagy, 1984) frameworks of therapy since children are almost completely dependent on adult caregivers for their growth and development. This ecological context includes the widening circle of psychosocial engagement such as family, neighbourhood, school, and the wider community.

In addition to this contextual model, child art therapy is predicated on the notion that art and play are essential domains of development, self-expression, and the possibilities of new realities and change (Landreth, 2012; Rubin, 2005). Daniel-Wariya identifies the 'magic circle' that is created in play as being "distinct in both space and time from the seriousness of the real world" (2019, p. 623). Within the play-state of the 'magic circle' that is created by the

DOI: 10.4324/9781003149538-7

therapist and child, emotional resonance is experienced by individuals, and ongoing resonance and meaning is carried between participating individuals even outside of the official play.

Art is a functional activity that carries meaning through its process and content that is critical for children's processing of thoughts, feelings, and reactions in therapy, developing coping strategies and a sense of self as agent (Waller, 2006). With younger children, developmentally informed use of sensory and kinesthetic art is needed to meet the therapeutic goals of self-regulation, focus, attention, and emotional awareness. Older children, who are already moving into symbolic processing and abstract thought, may use art to focus more on storytelling, narration, and symbolic discovery. With all age groups, metaphors within both the process of art making as well as the content of symbolic marks or images are observed and reflected as part of the therapy process (Buday, 2013), which focuses on the development of a 'self' that is increasingly flexible, adaptive, and capable of navigating life's challenges with reasonable and tolerable cognitive and emotional skills. Support for this development of an adaptive and coherent self must be embedded in work with parents/caregivers, teachers, and others who continually provide messages to children about their emotions, behaviours, and expectations (Regev & Snir, 2014).

Methodology

We create the frame of a 'third space' for therapy by setting the space, creating rituals for therapy, and by our attunement and reflection as therapists (Landreth, 2012). In a physical office, it is essential to designate an area as a child-centred space that is ready for exploration through art and play. When a child and their caregiver enter, they should feel like there is room for the child to connect and feel comfortable. The therapist's role is one of attunement, reflection, and limit-setting for safety as well as creating further art therapy interventions to engage coping and problem solving.

Basic Teletherapy Considerations

The switch to home spaces and computer-based contact has meant re-thinking how to continue to engage children, adolescents, and caregivers in the 'magic circle' of child art therapy. The first consideration is access to a computer or tablet, high-speed internet, and for the therapist to subscribe to a video conference platform that is stable and, for working in the US, is compliant with Health Insurance Portability and Accountability Act (HIPAA) rules. Clients consent to engage in teletherapy, which outlines confidentiality for both parties and contingency plans in case of failure with internet or computer access.

It may seem obvious that a child should be set up in a space that will allow for privacy when the adult caregiver leaves the room. In practice, however, this has been a tougher measure. Families find themselves in new and unique situations while we all navigate work from home, school from home, or other hybrid models. There are distractions that occur at home in ways that do not occur when visiting an office. In some cases, our set-up for privacy and the initial 10 minutes of caregiver/child time has had to be flexed to accommodate these factors. For younger children (ages four–six), the digital model has been challenging as their attention and focus is limited; therapy becomes more concentrated on solution-focused measures and caregiver/child interaction. Caregivers may become more involved in moving the child into a symbolic/creative act with the therapist coaching them in interactive engagement and reflection. With middle years children (6–12), leaving the child in front of the computer in a quiet space free from disruptions is easier, though some home situations may not allow for complete privacy. Establishing the sanctity of the 'magic circle' that carries between screens serves to not only create the space needed for a creative therapy process, but it also bolsters the sense of cordoning off distractions.

Likewise, having a variety of art and play tools easily accessible by the child is a challenge. We have found that creating a list of basic art supplies has been effective. At times, art supplies have been sent to a family for art experiences that are relevant to the goals. Working with found objects and other 'loose parts' (Figure 5.1), which might include pipe cleaners, toilet paper rolls, and other accessible materials, has become a routine part of the therapy practice. Additionally, utilizing the share-screen function or shareable websites (Table 5.1), which enable both therapist and child/adolescent to see the same screen while making art, has been a fun and useful find.

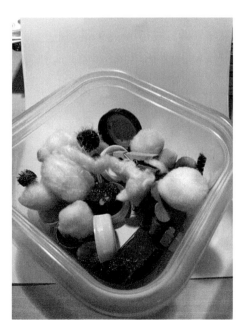

Figure 5.1 A Box of "Loose Parts"

Table 5.1 Digital Drawing Platforms

Platform	Features
Picmonkey; www.picmonkey.com	Photo editor and graphic design, collage, many visual effects
A Web Whiteboard (AWW); https://awwapp.com/#	Whiteboard with basic drawing capabilities, erasing, shapes, text, image upload and post-it notes; share and collaborate
Sketchbook; https://sketch.io/sketchpad/	Many drawing tools, colour choices, clipart, text and calligraphy, image upload, export as image or PDF
Adobe Creative Cloud Suite	Many creative and in-depth graphic, photo and drawing features, though there is a fee which can be more than many families want to spend on an additional platform for therapy
Google Jamboard in G-Suite (Google platforms)	Collaborative, can download images from a Google search or your computer, draw and erase, shape recognition tools, free

One of the hallmarks of social and emotional development through art therapy has been engaging children in shared art making. Using online tools has allowed us to continue to do this while children are in different spaces. Figure 5.2 shows the beginning prompts that participants in a group created together using the 'Yes, and' method from improv theatre.

Methodological Teletherapy Considerations

Digital screens and the home space of the child now frame creative processing within the 'magic circle.' Narrowing and expanding that frame are ways to accommodate the need for movement and kinesthetic engagement, mitigate distractions, and create new ways of connecting to the child in their space.

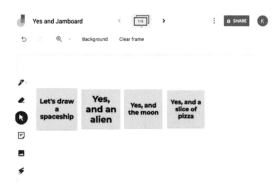

Figure 5.2 Group Art Therapy Jamboard Activity

The use of a Hoberman Sphere©—an engineered toy ball that expands and contracts with a series of hinges, often referred to in therapy circles as a 'breathing ball'—may concretely express ways that we expand into the space beyond our immediate computer screen to move, play, or make art, then come back to the near proximity of the video frame as the ball contracts. Using the ball for breathing is a great way to get a child and their caregiver grounded and focused on us since they often enter in a frazzled state as they transition from previous, home-based activity.

Waiting rooms sometimes serve as a transitional space before entering therapy, warranting other small gestures or rituals to help entice the young participant into a space with a different attention and intention. Maintaining the routine of having a caregiver check-in alongside the child is ideal. This, however, may be less focused or even difficult to accomplish if other demands are being placed on the caregiver. That said, the check-in creates a disruption, which focuses on the goals of therapy and helps the child move into a productive state for self-regulation and emotion tolerance.

Sharing screens for exploring current events, online images, or seek-and-finds, such as the intricate and fun illustrations of Gergely Dudas, may become new rituals that invite a time of settling and shared attention. I may allow a child to share their screen and lead the way into a particular interest so that they may assert some control as we settle in. Many public institutions have robust online offerings, and it can be fun to virtually visit zoos, museums, and places like NASA together. The Kansas City Zoo and The Nelson-Atkins Art Museum have released several videos throughout the pandemic of their penguins visiting the museum (and other places), which has been enjoyable to share and watch together.

Attunement and reflection are key therapeutic tools to helping a child become more self-aware, validated, and regulated; the drama needs to be enhanced for that to translate well into teletherapy. Additionally, our own movement to follow a child is limited within this new frame and we may miss an activity and subtle shifts in body language that we are used to catching in our in-person sessions. We may find ourselves wavering in unfamiliar territory without this valuable information and we may shift our focus more heavily into looking for more direct interaction and feedback as well as specific content within art and play.

Finding games and activities that can enable you to activate a client or settle them may help in finding new ways to attune and provide feedback for regulating emotions and behaviours. Scavenger hunts, character charades, freeze dance, and mindful breathing techniques are all useful tools to incorporate. For older children, reading guided meditations and including simple stretches or yoga poses may also serve to strengthen their body awareness in relation to their therapy goals associated with anxiety, depression, change, and stress. To tune into the sensory/motor and tactile qualities of art materials and art making processes, I have sent home recipes for making homemade dough with salt, flour, and water (Table 5.2), made sure that children and teens had access to newspaper for tearing and crumpling, and had caregivers create small bins of rice, beans, or other found objects for shaking, sifting, and then gluing and making things with.

Under office-based in-person circumstances, art and play may move somewhat fluidly within the space of the room and allotted time frame. In the digital landscape such movements between a variety of expressive activities may need more thought and intention. Breaking up the therapy time into segments that elicit information, allow for settling and sharing of attention, promote expression of invisible affect, create room for problem-solving and coping, and then transition away from the screen and back into day-to-day function requires more planning and tools 'on-hand.' While rituals can establish the start and end of sessions, the in-between time is trickier because emotion-laden material gets drummed up and exercised. We are without the physical aids that we are used to in the therapy room, necessitating more thoughtful consideration for how different activities can trigger a child and for how we utilize our toys, props, and dramatic command of voice and breath to bring awareness back to our shared space and attention.

Table 5.2 Salt Dough Recipe

Ingredients	Steps	
2 cups flour 1 cup salt 1 cup cold water	1)	Mix flour and salt together, slowly adding water a few tablespoons at time until smooth and easy to handle
	2)	Knead dough for 10 minutes then let rest for 20 minutes
	3)	Use 'as-is' or form into desired shapes, place on a cookie sheet and bake for 2 hours at 250°F

Case Vignettes

Adler (an alias used with permission) is a nine-year-old who I had been seeing in therapy for approximately five months before the pandemic necessitated shutdowns and work-from-home. His difficulty with maintaining attention, especially around emotion-laden material, and managing his bodily impulses had been apparent from the start. In my office, I could provide him with fidget toys and a clear set of expectations for the check-in time, which helped us to move through the rhythm of therapy sessions. Once we went to teletherapy, we had to re-establish routines, expectations, and consider how to help him manage his attention and body. While Adler is enthralled with computers and tech generally, helping him to focus on me on the other side of the screen became a struggle because of the enticing tabs and buttons. A great concern became discussing his challenges and needs related to handling his big emotions, working out social interactions and conflicts, and worry over his size, stature, and power within interpersonal relationships.

We started by having his mother set him up in a chair that cradled him, placing a blanket on his lap, and then pulling the computer in front with a rolling tray that could accommodate basic drawing supplies. During our check-in time, I would begin with the breathing ball to get his attention on me through the screen and to settle his body. We would then spend a few minutes reflecting on the challenges and triumphs from his week, allowing him to speak first before his mother would provide her oversight. Once his mother would step away, we would enter the shared space of the computer by sharing my screen and exploring something that would bring our attention together and offer a way to focus our eyes on a complex image that invited us to consider the action, story, or implied narrative.

After several weeks, I invited Adler, an antsy technology buff, to open a tab on his computer, share his screen with me and find a similarly interesting thing to share. This allowed him to be in control of letting me enter his world, while he selected something that could be shared, that offered a story he could relate to while also maintaining a boundary around what is expected in this digital landscape, i.e., he cannot go exploring endlessly. We would then move into art making as a reflective practice to help Adler identify and express his experiences and emotions as well as problem-solving. Figure 5.3 is an example of analog work that was saved as a screenshot.

We would end our sessions each week after Adler described his artwork. We would discuss any important elements of it together and then reflect on any coping strategies that came out of our session that could be important for him in the week ahead. Our final gesture for a goodbye is a wave to the camera with intentional eye contact directed at the camera, rather than looking somewhere on the screen to where the other person's face shows up. Eye contact is such an important concept in child social development that is easily obscured by screen-based teletherapy since our eyes are never actually aligned with the camera on the computer. This is certainly a concern for the use of videoconferencing in therapy that should be considered.

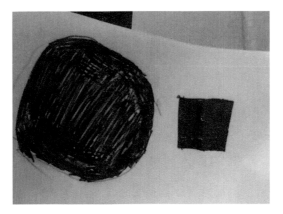

Figure 5.3 Adler's Drawing of His Emotions

The adolescents that I see have had very different needs and experiences in this time of pandemic shutdowns, alterations in school, and teletherapy. With adolescents, I have seen an increase in general anxiety, depression, social challenges, body image concerns, disordered eating behaviours, and lack of motivation or apathy. While they may be able to self-report much more effectively than a younger child, involving their caregivers in some conversations has been helpful to get a better picture on day-to-day functioning and to support effective adult-to-child communication at a time when everyone is feeling stressed.

Teens generally navigate the teletherapy world independently and may even have the appointment reminders texted to their own phones. Once we enter the teletherapy space, they are ready to engage on some level, usually having their own desks set for the experience. Many of my teens have taken to keeping visual journals where we have established creative prompts for drawing, painting, creating collages, or otherwise exploring their experiences, thoughts, feelings, and reactions. These journals have been used in-session as well as out-of-sessions for carryover into their weeks. Figure 5.4 shows images from a 16-year-old female client as she explored an alter ego character who emerged out of a scribble drawing. In talking about this curmudgeonly guy, we began to explore her sense of social isolation and subsequent anxiety in going outside while simultaneously longing for connection.

Digital platforms have been easier to share and teach to older children and adolescents, who are mostly already familiar with apps that enable photo editing, filtering, and adding stickers, emojis, and other elements. Helping them create mandalas through picmonkey© or other drawing platforms has led to many layered and visually rich images that express identity, feelings, as well as future-oriented plans and dreams. Teens have expressed enjoyment in playing with digital software alongside our use of their journals, as many platforms are available for tablets and phones, making them accessible throughout their day, providing a new activity for them on their phones instead of endless scrolling through social media.

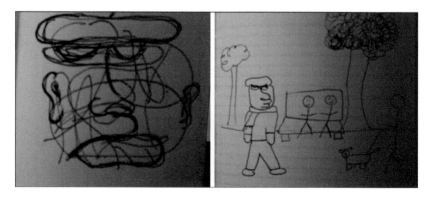

Figure 5.4 Scribble Drawing Turned into a Male Figure with a Beret

Challenges and Advantages

While making the radical shift to teletherapy was never part of my plan as a child and adolescent focused art therapist, I will say that the natural experiment that emerged has shown me some advantages to this format for service provision. First, I can see clients who may not otherwise be able to come to see me for many extenuating circumstances. For instance, I had worked with a young adolescent when she was a much younger child and lived in the city where I practice. Since that time, she and her family have moved out of the city. When new issues and needs arose a few months before the pandemic shutdowns, her parents called me looking for help. I saw her for a few sessions to assess the situation and tried to help her family find a therapist closer to home, to no avail as no one was taking new clients. Once the shutdowns occurred, it was easy for all of us to see that teletherapy was a viable option to continue therapy with me—someone who knew her history and the work we had done when she was much younger. In general, finding a therapist who specializes in young children is limited, even in my large, urban environment, and finding an art therapist is even trickier, making teletherapy an option for those who do not live anywhere near urban centres where therapists may be more available.

Additionally, some children and families are hesitant to come into an office to see someone about difficult or challenging issues. Being able to be in their own space may reduce this barrier and provide a more accessible path into treatment. Seeing a child's natural space and their own collection of toys and objects provides a valuable window into their world, imaginations, and general experiences. With this advantage comes the disadvantage of having the space be so familiar that the child may get distracted away from the focus on treatment. Likewise, other household distractions may disrupt the flow of therapy at times. Dogs, cats, and little siblings have invaded the therapy frame, causing minor and major distractions and, at times, also providing comfort or support.

Screen time and its impact on child and adolescent wellbeing is a consideration that falls under drawbacks to use of teletherapy with this population. Children and teens are already spending a good amount of time on screens for school, homework, and essential social connections, let alone their own investment in online gaming and other activities. While not all screen time is equal, the general passivity, distancing of interpersonal connection, eye strain, and other physical consequences link screen time to a number of negative outcomes, such as obesity, anxiety, depression, isolation, and poor sleep (Domingues-Montinari, 2017). Some children or adolescents have not found teletherapy comfortable during this time, and some families have identified that additional screen time was not appropriate for their child or adolescent. Furthermore, when engaging in teletherapy, we are at the mercy of internet connections and computer capacities. From time-to-time internet lags created pixelated images across screens, and connections have been dropped—something that becomes out of our control and frustrating. At the same time, on snow days or when a caregiver isn't feeling well, appointments might still be kept.

Finally, there is the issue of how to fully engage in art making, especially when the focus is on tactile, sensory, or dramatic arts to engage regulation at the body level. Adapting to the spaces that children and adolescents have has proven to be less of an issue than I originally thought, and art therapy treatment goals around improved awareness and communication, self-expression, and regulation of emotions have mostly been addressed through analog or screen-based art making processes. There continues to be some concern for being able to tune-in to the affective resonance in a fluid manner and adjust interventions as effectively through the screen. Additionally, I am limited to the tools at hand that a family has set-up for a child rather than the wide array of supplies, toys, and tools that I have at my office which has been developed over a 20-year career.

Conclusion

Art therapy centres the role of art for sensory-motor developmental functioning (Hinz, 2009; Kearns, 2004), expression, and communication (Silver, 2007), and as a source for developing adaptive and flexible coping strategies. Thus, art simultaneously buoys agency and autonomy and creates a 'third space' (Timm-Bottos & Reilly, 2015) where meaning is both conveyed and made between the therapist and child within the 'magic circle' of play. While I had no intention of exploring teletherapy as a regular part of my art therapy practice before the pandemic, it has become clear that there can be successful outcomes and unique art therapy experiences within the virtual, digital landscape.

This chapter highlights the processes and advantages as well as disadvantages of conducting tele art therapy with children and teens. In particular, factors around the home space regarding art materials and privacy have to be considered in order to lead therapeutic client sessions. The interaction between child and therapist through the screen reveals shortcomings, such as a lack of eye contact, but also a wider geographical reach to clients in locations with limited access to an art therapist. I think we need to continue to talk about the challenges and successes from this time of experimentation during the pandemic and consider how we can research best practices and efficacy across this service delivery platform as tele art therapy moves forward.

References

Boszmorenyi-Nagy, I. (1984). *Invisible loyalties: Reciprocity in intergenerational family therapy* (2nd edition). New York: Harper & Row.

Buday, K. M. (2013). Engage, empower, and enlighten: Art therapy and image making in hospice care. *Progress in Palliative Care, 21*(2), 83–88. https://doi.org/10.1179/1743291X13Y.0000000050.

Choudry, R., & Keane, C. (2021). *Art therapy during a mental health crisis: Coronavirus pandemic impact report*. American Art Therapy Association. https://arttherapy.org/up load/Art-Therapy-Coronavirus-Impact-Report.pdf.

Daniel-Wariya, J. (2019). Rhetorical strategy and creative methodology: Revisiting Homo Ludens. *Games and Culture, 14*(6). https://doi.org/10.1177/1555412017721085.

Domingues-Montinari, S. (2017). Clinical and psychological effects of excessive screen time. *Journal of Pediatrics and Child Health, 53*, 333–338. https://doi.org/10.1111/jpc.13462.

Gerlitz, Y., Regev, D., & Snir, S. (2020). A relational approach to art therapy. *The Arts in Psychotherapy, 68*, 101644. https://doi.org/10.1016/j.aip.2020.101644.

Hinz, L. (2009). *Expressive arts therapies continuum: A framework for using art in therapy.* New York: Routledge.

Kearns, D. (2004). Art therapy with a child experiencing sensory integration difficulty. *Art Therapy: Journal of the American Art Therapy Association, 21*(2), 95–101.

Landreth, G. (2012). *Play therapy: The art of the relationship.* New York: Routledge.

Levy, C. E., Spooner, H., Lee, J. B., Sonke, J., Myers, K., & Snow, E. (2018). Tele-health-based creative arts therapy: Transforming mental health and rehabilitation care for rural veterans. *The Arts in Psychotherapy, 57*, 20–26. https://doi.org/10.1016/j.aip.2017.08.010.

Ray, D. C. (2018). The child and the counselor: Relational humanism in the playroom and beyond. *Journal of Humanistic Counseling, 58*, 68–82. https://doi.org/10.1002/johc.12090.

Regev, D., & Snir, S. (2014). Working with parents in parent-child art psychotherapy. *The Arts in Psychotherapy, 41*, 511–518. https://dx.doi.org/10.1016/j.aip.2014.10.001.

Rubin, J. (2005). *Child art therapy, 25th Anniversary Edition.* New York: Wiley.

Silver, R. (2007). *The Silver drawing test and draw a story, assessing depression, aggression, and cognitive skills.* New York: Routledge.

Spivak, S., Spivak, A., Cullen, B, Meuchel, J., Johnston, D., Chernow, R., Green, C., & Mojtabai, R. (2020). Telepsychiatry in US mental health facilities, 2010–2017. *Psychiatric Services, 72*, 121–127. https://doi.org/10.1176/appi.ps.201900261.

Timm-Bottos, J., & Reilly, R. C. (2015). Learning in third spaces: Community art studio as storefront university classroom. *American Journal of Community Psychology, 55*, 102–114. doi:10.1007/s10464-014-9688-5.

Waller, D. (2006). Art therapy for children: How it leads to change. *Clinical Child Psychology and Psychiatry, 11*(2), 271–282. https://doi.org/10.1177/1359104506061419.

6 Reaching City Youth with an Online Summer Arts Workshop in Los Angeles

Jessica Bianchi and Amber Cromwell

Introduction

The Summer Arts Workshop (SAW) is a community-based art therapy program with a social justice focus. It has been offered through the Helen B. Landgarten (HBL) Art Therapy Clinic at Loyola Marymount University (LMU) since 2007 in partnership with Dolores Mission School in Boyle Heights, a historically under-resourced part of East Los Angeles. In 2020, due to the COVID-19 pandemic and stay-at-home orders in Los Angeles, the SAW leadership team adapted the workshop to an online format. We took advantage of the online format to extend the reach of the workshop to several school sites in marginalized communities in Los Angeles County, including a juvenile hall high school, which is a prison for youth in a state youth detention centre. The greatest challenge in adapting to an online format was preserving the core component of the workshop: building trust and healthy attachments through expressive art making. We overcame this and other challenges and succeeded in providing connecting experiences for participants and facilitators during a time of social isolation and collective anxiety.

History and Development of the Summer Arts Workshop

"I feel like I can take off my mask and be accepted for who I am, and this makes me want to keep trying new things and meet new people." These are the words of 11-year-old Paty Hernandez in 2007 after her first year of participating in SAW. Paty is now in her twenties working as a civil engineer, the first in her family to graduate from college. Fourteen years later, she continues to play a crucial role in the leadership of SAW.

SAW began as an arts initiative sponsored by Loyola Marymount University's (LMU) College of Communication and Fine Arts (CFA) called Arts Pro Bono. This pilot program was facilitated by senior faculty members in the MFT/Art Therapy Department in partnership with Dolores Mission School. Initial funding came from a small, private donation that increased over the years and eventually allowed the program to charter a bus to pick up youth at Dolores Mission School and shuttle them across Los Angeles to the university every day for a week in the summer.

DOI: 10.4324/9781003149538-8

Throughout the week, the youth engage in cumulative multimedia art making that culminates in a final exhibition for friends, family, and university personnel. The youth are supported by graduate student trainees from the MFT/Art Therapy Department, who provide a warm and supportive foundation. The program promotes inquiry, problem-solving, and compassionate exploration of oneself, others, relationships, culture, and perceived place within the community. Art making is used to explore and promote positive cultural identity formation amongst youth, many of whom are first-generation Americans impacted by adversity, poverty, gang violence, and family displacement.

Dolores Mission is a transitional kindergarten through 8th-grade school that serves approximately 260 children. The student population is 97% Latinx, with 60% of the students classified as English Language Learners. Seventy-five percent of the families live below the federal poverty level, despite one or both parents working full-time (Dolores Mission School, n.d.). Once the poorest mission in Los Angeles, the school is now a beacon of light, colour, and laughter despite the impact of extremely high rates of violence and adversity.

One youth asked one of our graduate student mentors, "I don't know why you guys chose me to join the program. I'm such a troublemaker." The mentor responded, "Well, you might be, but here you're an art maker." This interaction is an example of how SAW is grounded in Positive Youth Development Theory (PYD), which aims to identify and develop strength-based qualities in youth, such as leadership, motivation, compassion, creativity, and resilience, rather than focusing on calling out negative or maladaptive behavior, such as oppositional defiance, attention deficit, and negative attention-seeking (Damon, 2004). Popular discourse holds that youth can pose serious harm to self and others and "must be straightened out" before problems arise (Damon, 2004, p. 14). This negative interpretation of young people, and especially young people of colour, has become a well-known view of adolescents. News media coverage has increasingly portrayed youth as negative (Kwon, 2006). This stereotype can have a severely damaging impact on adolescents who internalize these negative associations. PYD suggests that helping young people identify their strengths through art making can protect against adverse development (Gillham et al., 2002).

In the early years of SAW, many of the youth participants asked to continue in the program even after they had graduated from middle school. This prompted us to shift our programming to meet this need. Middle-school participants can now become 'junior mentors,' and junior mentors have the opportunity to become hired as paid 'senior mentors' when they turn 18 years old.

In addition to providing multiple opportunities for youth to explore and build positive identity and community bonds, SAW provides a rich training experience for graduate art therapy students. They can experience a type of art therapy service that is community-focused and meets clients in their own space, both figuratively and metaphorically.

Bianchi and Blueskyes (2007) evaluated the first Summer Arts Workshop and explored emergent themes, including opportunities to develop self-esteem, positive risk-taking, and increased sense of belonging through the use of therapeutic art making. Further research followed with Jones (2009), who was interested in how SAW provides a safe space for Latinx adolescent youth to explore identity and engage in vital cultural identity exploration, often in the context of immigration stressors. Cromwell and Patch (2004) continued exploring the significance of empathy and positive attachment for some of the original participants, which was expanded by Melendez (2012), who studied two individuals who started as youth participants, became junior mentors, and eventually became paid senior mentors.

Expansion to Online Programming at Dolores Mission

Given our dedication to SAW and its role in serving Dolores Mission and LMU, we knew in May 2020 that it would be particularly important for youth to come together in SAW to process the stress and anxiety brought on by the pandemic and social unrest surrounding George Floyd's murder. With nation-wide closures and lockdowns, the program would have to be an online pro-gram, rather than in person. Thus, we began figuring out how to maintain integral pieces of the program: the safety felt by the youth (both physical and emotional), the engaging and interactive process of the art making, and the magic that happens as a result of relationship and community building.

We knew there could be problems with access to technology as well as privacy, legal, and connectivity issues. A therapist might have to choose between seeing the clients' facial expressions or their art process, which could impede authentic relationship building. However, research suggested that tele-art therapy could be an effective and adaptable tool and create moments of intimacy with the opportunity to virtually enter a person's home (Collie & Cubranic, 2002; Collie et al., 2006; Levy et al., 2018; Spooner et al., 2019).

We decided to use *all* of the art disciplines in this year's program—not only visual art, but music, movement, and performance art, too—to provide addi-tional kinesthetic stimulation. Furthermore, we were unsure whether or not we could get visual art supplies to all the youth and, thus, did not want to only rely on visual art activities alone.

Project Theme

With civil uprising and a pandemic strongly impacting the Dolores Mission community, we knew that we wanted a curriculum centred on advocacy, allyship, and empowerment. Spooner et al. (2019) have claimed that telehealth can bridge gaps of access for people in marginalized communities and provide opportunities to express their resiliency and amplify their voices, especially in times of societal stress. Accordingly, our project theme was "Amplify: How can we use our art to make louder the voices that need to be heard, including our own?" In order to explore this theme in a developmentally and culturally engaging way, we decided that we would create a collaborative music video that would integrate visual art, music, and movement.

Objectives

When meeting in-person during the previous years, we created opportunities for abstract and critical thinking, problem solving, relationship building, and perspective taking. If we wanted to maintain these objectives and the integrity of the SAW program online, we needed to learn how to create a space for empathy, a pillar of what makes this program so special. Furthermore, we wanted to have a good understanding of how to use the technology in an elevated and dynamic way and explore how we could get quality mark making materials to each individual household.

Curriculum Development

Typically, we have meetings with our graduate students to develop the curriculum, but this year we decided to include our guest teaching artists and therefore scheduled a series of Zoom meetings for planning. In adapting our curriculum to an online platform, we wanted to mirror the same approach we use when we are in person. For five days, students learn new skills every day and are exposed to new art techniques to support creation of intentional art focused on positive cultural identity development. The mentors model the art process and help students understand the concepts relating to the overarching theme by asking questions and encouraging deeper exploration. We layer our lessons; starting first with exploration of personal characteristics, we open to cultural factors within family and community structures, and culminate with a broadened understanding of community and society. In order to do this, we name a question of the day. Each day's icebreakers, games, art interventions, and reflections are aimed at helping the participant answer that question for themselves. By days four and five, participants have created individual and collaborative art pieces that answer these questions and elicit further conversations that they can bring to their community. The week culminates with a virtual ceremony where the work is displayed in a professional manner and all of our participants receive special awards.

The following table 6.1 presents the final online curriculum showing the question of the day, objective for the day, and creative tools that would be used to meet the day's objective.

Program Implementation Strategies

During our typical in-person week, we have a large whiteboard where we display the question of the day and the schedule of events. This strategy is an important part of a trauma-informed approach in order to create consistency and safety in our space. We decided to replicate this strategy for the online platform and used Google Slides to create a virtual bulletin board that would act as our home base.

Table 6.1 SAW Online Curriculum

	Question of the day	Objective	Creative tools
Day 1	What's going on? *(using art as a way to check-in with ourselves)*	Students will seek inspiration from artists	• Zoom • *word cloud to high-light observations
Day 2	Community *(using art to imagine a world of justice for all)*	Explore personal and ideal spaces	• GarageBand • developing choreography
Day 3	Stand up/take a knee *(using bodies to make art)*	Recognize the power of using art to stand up for important things	• Zoom recordings • photos
Day 4	Amplify *(using art to make perspectives louder and more visible)*	Using elements of art to convey a message	• community board
Day 5	Wake up *(call the community to action)*	Sharing art in a collective space	• Zoom space for virtual celebration • YouTube to share video

Note: Curriculum development credit: A. Cromwell, J. Bianchi, L. Butler, M. Bogdanow, and M. Herrera.
*A word cloud is a collection, or cluster, or words depicted in different sizes. There are many free generators that you can find by simply typing word cloud in a search engine.

We called it the Community Board (Figure 6.1). It was available to any of the participants outside of our workshop hours so that they could go back and refer to some of the content we shared and have a look at what is in store for them the next day. The Community Board had links to inspirational videos and artist works. If anyone lost the connection to our Zoom call, they would have the contact information for directors and the Zoom link to join again. Additionally, we created slides titled "Meet the Mentors" with a little blurb about each graduate student and teaching artist to facilitate the mentor–mentee relationship.

Another strategy that we typically implement from a trauma-informed model is having an element of choice to allow participants to feel a sense of control and agency in the space. We were able to do this online by leaving it up to the participants to turn on their cameras or their microphones. In addition, we created breakout rooms in Zoom where participants had the option of choosing which art discipline they preferred for the week: music, movement, or lyric writing. Lastly, we ended each day with hands-on art making using the physical art materials that we had delivered or mailed to them. During this time, we modelled a technique and then encouraged the youth to choose how they wanted to explore their personal connections to the question of the day.

Audio and video recordings of sounds, movements, and visual art were made every step of the way so that the process itself became the footage for

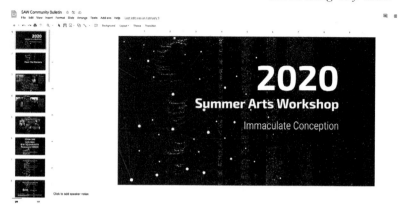

Figure 6.1 Community Board

the final music video. The graduate student mentors played a pivotal role in modelling the art process, encouraging participants through the chat, and staying focused and present with participants every step of the way. Several mentors noted that the experience was an opportunity to not only increase their familiarity with delivering art therapy online, but to also work with new populations. Furthermore, the experience allowed them to deepen their relationships with their graduate student peers while enduring their own isolation.

Program Delivery to Dolores Mission School

In June and July of 2020, we implemented our newly adapted virtual SAW to 16 middle school students from Dolores Mission School. We encountered many challenges and opportunities to adapt and readjust our approach to providing our first online SAW. On day one, we observed low energy from participants and facilitators, perhaps due to the newness of being in a virtual space. It was difficult to read body language and attune with the participants because many had their cameras off. We realized that the phrase we often use in therapy, "meet them where they are at," had new layers of meaning in relation to technology.

Prior to the workshop, we had made every effort to mail or hand-deliver art materials to each of the participants, but despite these efforts, there were still some participants that reported they didn't have the materials on hand. With no art materials, we had to get creative and encourage participants to use what was available. One student made art with sticky notes; another used lipstick. Additionally, we had participants that were accessing Zoom using different devices, such as iPhones, laptops, iPads, and Chromebooks. Each of these devices had different functionality, and we had to become well versed in how to direct participants to access Zoom and the other programs and applications we used.

There were also cultural and developmental factors that arose. For example, one participant was taking care of his younger sibling and was frequently in and out of the screen tending to the needs of his brother. Additionally, in our efforts to encourage participants to turn their video on, we also had to be sensitive to the fact that many participants might be experiencing shame about their home environments. Another participant had such limited space in his home that he opted to create art outside despite the intense summer heat. With regards to the movement aspect of the workshop, asking adolescents to dance is always high risk due to typical self-consciousness around the body. Thus, there were initially a lot of cameras off in the movement groups. One of our attempts to address these issues was to be very slow and thoughtful. We slowed down movement activities and focused movement on parts of the body that the participants appeared to be more comfortable sharing—for example, their hands. We also assigned mentors to different students so they could consistently reach out to them by chat throughout the week and have more of a personal one-on-one conversation about any of the above-mentioned issues in order to support and gently invite participation.

The following images, Figures 6.2, 6.3, 6.4, and 6.5, show some of the processes and results, highlighting the success of the program.

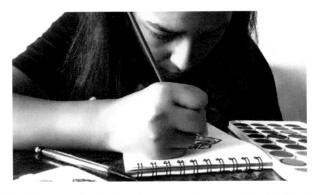

Figure 6.2 Participant in Art Making Process as Shown in Wake Up Music Video

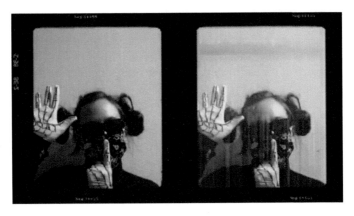

Figure 6.3 SAW Participant Explores Storytelling through Imagery

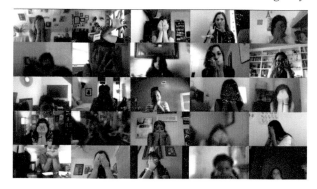

Figure 6.4 SAW Participants Explore How to Evoke Feelings through Body Movement

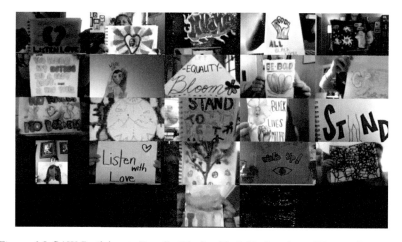

Figure 6.5 SAW Participants Proudly Display Their Exploration of Protest Art

Adaptations at the Juvenile Hall High School

In May 2020, the HBL Art Therapy Clinic was strengthening its partnership with a juvenile hall high school in a state-funded youth detention centre just north of downtown Los Angeles. Due to the previous success of the virtual SAW at Dolores Mission and abundant art therapy graduate student participation, we decided to offer this program for the first time to this school. It was an opportunity that emerged because of the new online aspect of the program, which did not require us to physically enter the juvenile hall.

The high school serves approximately 200 6th–12th grade students in East Los Angeles, 19% female-presenting and 81% male-presenting. Ninety-six percent of the students are from a minority ethnic background: 55% Latinx, 38% Black, 4% White, 1% Asian, 0.5% American Indian/Alaskan Native, and 0.5% two or more races. Almost all were identified as economically disadvantaged and eligible for the Free Lunch Program, a federally assisted meal program. The school has an 8% graduation rate.

The principal informed us of the many protocols that we might expect from the state probation department ('Probation'), which protects the legal and ethical rights of the youth who are wards of the state. Due to confidentiality issues for online programming, our mentor team was not permitted to see the faces of the youth on the computer screen. "Okay, we can be creative," responded the team. "We'll have the youth angle their cameras onto their art and they can be really expressive using their hands." The team revised the original Amplify music video curriculum to be more focused on recording hand gestures, sounds, and visual imagery for the music video.

A follow-up meeting with the principal occurred several weeks later. "So listen," he said, "I spoke with Probation and unfortunately, due to increased confidentiality requirements, you won't be able to take screenshots or record any of the hand gestures or art in your sessions with the students."

"Okay. Got it," replied the team. We went back to the drawing board and adapted the program to be a zine project instead of a music video. Zines have historically been a form of social justice art wherein the goal is to self-produce a visual art piece that communicates or educates on a certain topic. Each individual youth would create their own zine, using different visual art materials and processes on each page about the daily question. They could combine their art to create a collaborative zine that the graduate student mentors would consolidate, print, and mail to the juvenile high school.

The team was feeling confident about the adaptations and enthusiastically reported the progress to the principal. "More news from Probation," he said. "In order to provide the utmost protection for the youth, we have been told that the participants will not be permitted to have their cameras on at all during the workshop. But my teaching staff is dedicated to helping make this program really meaningful for the youth. Maybe we can take pictures of the kids' art and send them to you at the end of each session?" he offered.

We continued to experience requirements from probation that prompted us to further adapt the program. Our workshop had to move from a Zoom platform to Microsoft Teams, a different online meeting platform that was approved for student usage by Probation. This meant that the digital art making applications we had used in our original online plan would not be accessible to our juvenile hall participants. Instead, only physical art materials would be used to create art that we wouldn't be able to see.

In addition to addressing technology, privacy, legal, and connectivity issues, we had to reconsider the art therapists' reliance on witnessing clients' art making as well as art products in the process of art therapy (Levy et al., 2018; Spooner et al., 2019). We recognized that, without high-quality images in front of them, the mentors were going to have to rely heavily on client verbal descriptions and perhaps miss subtle details, something documented by Levy et al. in a 2018 study of telecommunication-based creative arts therapy with

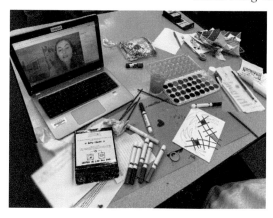

Figure 6.6 Image of High School Participant Point of View

veterans. Nonetheless, we moved forward with the assurance of resources, support, and technical assistance from the juvenile high school staff.

The principal and his staff engaged in consistent feedback with our team via text and email throughout the week. Text communication between the principal and our project coordinator included the exchange of images for the completed zine, where it was his task to take photographs of the participant artwork each day after the session.

The principal expressed his appreciation about how well things were going. He acknowledged how fast the art therapy graduate students were able to build rapport with the youth. In reflection, he stated that students in juvenile hall are often let down by the adult figures in their lives and are typically cautious of trusting adults. However, he observed his students build enough rapport with the mentors to the point where they appeared to feel "vulnerable." He continued to say that he believed the distance created through teletherapy allowed the youth to feel more comfortable with the "strangers"—the art therapy graduate student mentors—and allowed them "entrance" into their living space.

Limited in their ability to see the participants, their art, or their art process, the mentors worked to find other ways to engage and connect with the youth. Early in the week, one of the mentors experimented with music, sharing personal music preferences and encouraging the youth to do the same. This connection prompted more interaction through the chat option in Teams. With the only agenda being an authentic desire to hear what the youth participants wanted to say and know who they were, relationships started to grow between the mentors and participants. Not being able to see the participants' artwork appeared to allow for a different kind of connection, one in which the participant was in control. A facilitator commented on how they learned to look past the audio-only barrier and, by the end, viewed it as an opportunity to shed biases and see through participants' eyes.

Figure 6.7 is an artist's recreation of one of the student works. It wasn't until after the day's workshop that the principal would send images of the artwork to

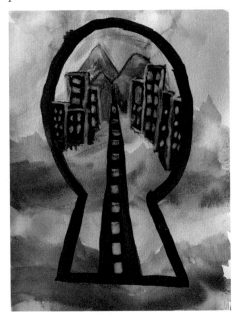

Figure 6.7 Recreation of Juvenile High School Student Art, Watercolour on Paper

our team; therefore, the mentors had to rely on their imagination to picture the art being described to them. In reflection during supervision, one of our mentors expressed how profound this experience was, noting that it removed any opportunity to project onto the image, but rather hear and connect with the words of the student. For instance, the student described her art (Figure 6.7 above) as expressing her desire to find the key to leave her problems behind and get out of Los Angeles. It was interesting for our mentors to have an idea in their minds of the image being described and to then be given the opportunity to see the image itself after the workshop. Our graduate students shared that it made them feel very connected to the message and the theme behind the imagery.

Interestingly, the opportunity to deepen relationships trickled down to the relationships between participants and their teachers as well as participants and their probation officers. Initially, our mentors found it challenging to provide art therapy services while the participants' classroom teachers were present. The mentors had to field well-intentioned comments from non-clinical adults, such as "That's so pretty!," which might derail a participant's authentic expression. It appeared, however, that the encouragement to express their thoughts, ideas, and feelings around an evocative and personally relevant topic became an opportunity for participants to feel a sense of agency in an environment where they may have felt little. The principal commented that what stood out the most to him was how the participants' exploration through the art allowed them to be vulnerable and then subsequently be praised and accepted for that vulnerability. In addition, he described that the participants' ability to create something that they valued, thus lowering their usual defenses, allowed the teachers and staff to see the kids in a different way. He reflected that the teachers and staff saw new strengths and skills that had gone unseen before, speaking to the program's desire to address positive youth development. The principal commented that Probation was curious and interested in seeing what the participants were creating and this appeared to shift the relationship dynamic, where probation officers were interacting with the youth in a curious way versus relaying orders and restrictions.

At the ceremony at the end of the week, we usually acknowledge the relationship between senior mentors and their one or two youth participants by having the adult mentor give that particular student their certificate and say something personal about them and their process. In order to replicate this experience in our virtual program, we asked the principal if we could have teachers and staff present during the culminating ceremony. He was so enthusiastic about the work and content created by the youth that he wanted to invite not only teachers and staff, but other members of his leadership team, as well as members from the probation department. He highlighted that there was potential to use the zines as a means to communicate aspects of the participants' recovery to the probation court, including their judge, thereby helping improve the terms of their incarceration.

During the ceremony, LMU guests/facilitators were displayed on a big screen in a community room. While we couldn't see anyone in the room, we could hear the celebration and the festive tone. When it came time to say goodbye, we heard some heartfelt and warm thank yous, and then our job was done.

Conclusion

This chapter shows how teletherapy can bridge gaps of access, particularly for marginalized populations. The Helen B. Landgarten Art Therapy Clinic at Loyola

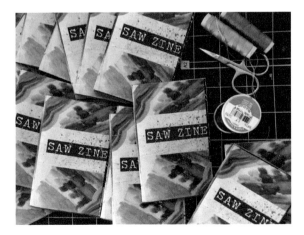

Figure 6.8 Completed Zines from Juvenile Hall

Marymount University implemented a positive youth development program in the form of Summer Arts Workshops with the objectives of providing opportunities for critical thinking, problem-solving, relationship building, and perspective-taking. The program was delivered to Dolores Mission school, culminating in a student-created music video, and changed to a zine format for delivery at a juvenile hall high school. Both art making projects included an element of choice for the participants and served to empower them as they showed vulnerability and found strength through these personal expressions.

Although telecommunication tools allowed us to access the population at juvenile hall for the first time, the online format brought challenging limitations that we had to overcome, such as not being able to see the students or the art because cameras had to stay turned off for confidentiality reasons. This put the participants in control, which provided the therapists with the opportunity to see the art through the participants' eyes. The principal revealed that he saw the youth express deeper parts of themselves in the art, which was different from the defenses he usually observed. The youth participants seemed strengthened to take positive risks in their art process, be vulnerable in their expressions, and receive praise for their efforts.

In both workshops, the participants were able to amplify their voices and call their community to listen. Through the process of expanding technology and adapting to the needs of different populations, our efforts to create a safe space for youth to express themselves appeared incredibly successful.

References

Bianchi, J., & Blueskyes, O. (2007). *Community arts outreach with los income urban Latino adolescents.* [Unpublished doctoral dissertation/master's thesis] Loyola Marymount University.

Collie, K., & Cubranic, D. (2002). Computer-supported distance art therapy: A focus on traumatic illness. *Journal of Technology in Human Services, 20*(1–2), 155–171.

Collie, K., Bottorff, J. L., Long, B. C., & Conati, C. (2006). Distance art groups for women with breast cancer: Guidelines and recommendations. *Supportive Care in Cancer, 14*(8), 849–858.

Cromwell, A., & Patch, A. (2004). *Attachment, empathy, and mentorship in a community arts workshop with adolescents.* [Unpublished doctoral dissertation/master's thesis] Loyola Marymount University.

Damon, W. (2004). What is positive youth development? *Annals of the American Academy of Political and Social Science, 591,* 13–24.

Dolores Mission School. (n.d.). *School History.* https://doloresmissionschool.org/school-history.

Gillham, J. E., Reivich K., & Shatte, A. (2002). Positive youth development, prevention, and positive psychology: Commentary on positive youth development in the United States. *Prevention and Treatment, 5*(18).

Kwon, S. A. (2006). Youth of color organizing for juvenile justice. In S. Ginwright, p. Noguera, & J. Cammarota (Eds.), *Beyond resistance: Youth activism and community change: New democratic possibilities for policy and practice* (pp. 215–228). New York: Routledge Press.

Jones, C. M. (2009). *Latino adolescent development through community arts outreach.* [Unpublished doctoral dissertation/master's thesis] Loyola Marymount University.

Levy, C. E., Spooner, H., Lee, J. B., Sonke, J., Meyers, K., & Snow, E. (2018). Telehealth-based creative arts therapy: Transforming mental health and rehabilitation care for rural veterans. *The Arts in Psychotherapy, 57*(1), 20–26. doi: https://doi.org/10.1016/j.aip.2017.08.010.

Melendez, A. (2012). *The lived experience of mentorship.* [Unpublished doctoral dissertation/master's thesis] Loyola Marymount University.

Spooner, H., Lee, J. B., Langston, D. G., Sonke, J., Myers, K. J., & Levy, C. E. (2019). Using distance technology to deliver the creative arts therapies to veterans: Case studies in art, dance/movement and music therapy. *The Arts in Psychotherapy, 62*(1), 12–18. doi: https://doi.org/10.1016/j.aip.2018.11.012.

7 The Screen as a Stage

Artistic Methods for Group Arts-Based Therapy via Zoom

Ronen Berger

Prologue

Like many art therapists, I had not conducted art therapy online prior to the pandemic and the lockdowns and isolations that followed. As I taught art therapy and supervised art therapists during this period, I explored different ways of using the screen artistically for arts-based therapy. The growing isolation and loneliness that I came across emphasized the need for specific group and community virtual art therapy methods.

During this process, I became aware of many differences between the kind of work that takes place in face-to-face settings and encounters that take place in virtual space. I recognized the impact on issues such as group space, relationships, authority, creativity, privacy, and ethics, as well as for methods used in general and in group work in particular (Berger & Liber, 2021; Collie & Čubranić, 1999; Shuper-Engelhard & Furlager, 2020).

In my practice, I try to maintain an *art as therapy* orientation and work mainly via the artistic process and less through verbal conversations. This can be a challenge on the Zoom videoconferencing platform, where audio is an essential part of the communication. Experimenting in individual and group settings with clients, students, and supervisees helped me use the screen as a creative platform—a stage for artistic presentations.

This chapter presents concepts and methods supporting virtual arts-based therapy to develop client coping skills, resilience, depression support, and personal growth. Methods include synchronous therapist-led group work on Zoom and asynchronous client participation on online platforms, such as, Google Drive and Padlet. The chapter will conclude with thoughts about further development of practice, research, supervision, and training.

Virtual Space, Virtual Dynamics—Meanings and Implementations for Group Work

The shift from a physical group, organized and maintained by the therapist, into an online collective space creates a unique therapeutic environment. The therapist and group members are all present on screen in the here and now and

DOI: 10.4324/9781003149538-9

able to see and hear each other while forming and holding a collective group space. At the same time, they may be physically separated.

There are several possible setups for this encounter:

- The most common setup occurs when the therapist and each participant is located alone in a different location while communicating virtually through their screen.
- The therapist is located away from the group and the group members are able to communicate and create together in one physical space. In this case, the therapist is present virtually—for example, in residential care settings or boarding schools.
- The therapist is located alone and there are multiple groups of participants who only share the same physical spaces within each group, such as small groups of clients meeting locally in several remote communities and connecting virtually with the other groups as well as the art therapist.

Regarding the concepts of therapeutic space and encounter space, or space in which therapy happens, the varying possibilities of session formats listed above need distinct adaptations. For example, in the second and third setups, some participants share the same physical spaces and can participate collectively with the materials. They can form a composition that includes physical touch and joint sculpture or collaborations in space that cannot be performed through videoconferencing, such as in the first setup. The use of virtual spaces and the physical absence of the therapist changes the basic concepts of relationships and group dynamics.

For example, Zoom, like other videoconferencing platforms, randomly chooses where each participant will be located on the screen and adjacent to whom. Moreover, the software's algorithm is programmed so that each participant is located next to the host (facilitator) on each participant's screen. Consequently, the facilitator and participants will have a different view of the group's appearance, which affects group space, group mapping, and social interaction; in other words, transforming the collective physical space of encounter into a digital representation made up of squares on a screen changes our perception of one another, relationships within the group, and communication styles. We cannot enter or exit the other's personal physical space, nor touch or move their bodies.

This aspect also influences collective artistic work and the nature of the collaborative creative space. Using shared digital boards, we can draw together; using editing apps, we can organize and create collective digital exhibitions. Nevertheless, these expressions of the creative process and its meaning are experientially and artistically different from the traditional group creative process as they lack the physical presence that is shared with other group members. Thus, some clients may not feel as close to each other in order to collaborate as deeply. Furthermore, the art materials and the products will be presented in a two-dimensional perspective and lack depth, smell, and touch for other group members.

The use of the virtual space influences the roles available for participants as well as their dynamics. For example, participants who were accustomed to assuming a caretaker role by providing refreshments or taking care of the room's organization might find that the role no longer exists. On the other hand, participants equipped with technological knowledge regarding the internet, Zoom, and other applications can help participants and facilitators resolve difficulties and find a new role in the group.

The divergences between physical and virtual therapeutic encounters can make the same group appear differently in the two settings. The therapist should keep this situation in mind when planning and facilitating the group. Special consideration should be given to hybrid situations when the process includes a mixture of physical encounters and digital ones as well as shifts between the three kinds of encounters that were presented earlier. It is pertinent that we explore the meanings of these transitions and examine what will best suit the specific group: a physical setting, a virtual setting, or a combination of the two. The therapist may choose to involve the group in a discussion of the issue, to hear their participants' voices, and then decide what suits best that particular group.

Control, Authority, and Power

As in a non-virtual setting, the therapist in a videoconferencing arts-based group fills the role of an authority presence. The role of Host offers many empowering features, including the creation of the meeting and deciding who may join, and when. The role of Co-Host entails similar features, but it is up to the discretion of the therapist to select a participant as Co-Host or leave the position unassigned. The therapist, as Host, has the ability to control aspects of participation, including muting individual microphones, removing people from the call, and having the power to record and save the meeting. The Host is also the only participant who can move among breakout rooms and close them. These Zoom capabilities grant therapists an element of control different from those available in classic therapy encounters. Since the tools' influence and meaning on group dynamics and participants' experience can be dramatic, it is advised to pay attention to how they are used.

At the same time, videoconferencing gives participants new and different ways to express feelings and involvement in the sessions. For instance, participants can turn off their cameras, use the chat, leave the session, or join it later, thus changing the group matrix and atmosphere. These digital expressions can be addressed as new forms of "acting out" or "resistance" and raise dilemmas for therapists seeking to react appropriately. For example, is it appropriate and ethical to ask or insist that participants turn on their cameras? How should refusals be handled? Should therapists accede to a participant's request to remain unseen or only partially visible, or should they insist that participants turn on their cameras and be seen in the encounter as a prerequisite for participation in a similar way to a physical encounter?

Other questions relate to the therapist's choices as an authority figure. For example, what size group should be allowed? Should it be limited to the number of participants that can be seen on one screen, or could it include a larger number—enough to fill more than one screen, preventing the therapist from seeing everyone simultaneously? Or should the therapist be encouraged to obtain large screens for a better view?

Traditionally, art therapy occurs in the therapist's clinic or studio, providing participants with a safe and private physical space to share and explore personal issues. Being detached from their everyday reality establishes a kind of sacred space for clients (Pendzik, 1994). Carrying out virtual therapeutic encounters undermines this fundamental belief. Regarding this shift, I recommend starting the session with some form of transitional ritual. A meditation or mindfulness activity can be used, such as closing the eyes and taking a few breaths, drawing a picture, playing music, dancing, or voicing out a monologue.

Using Technology to Improve Therapy

Using video conversations for therapy allows us to incorporate different digital elements from our personal devices in the sessions. This includes sharing music, videos, photos, and text. Utilizing recordings and screen captures of meetings are possible interventions. These can be altered through digital means and elements of them can be used by the therapist and client.

The therapist and group members can share a song or video clip to present an artistic medium or technique relevant to a participant's work to inspire and support the process of artistic creation. The therapist can find images, songs, and clips online to be used as artistic responses, echoing back to the client in symbolic and artistic manners. Similarly, participants can use the media to share elements from their world with the therapist and other group members. Incorporating these technologies into arts-based therapy enriches the experience.

A variety of programs and browser-based applications can be used for online editing and sharing, such as Padlet, which enables the creation of an artistic group presentation and dialogue between members. These technologies can be used in synchronous work during sessions as well as for asynchronous work after and between meetings. Taking a screenshot can capture and save on-screen images to a device and allows the therapist to send them to participants. These elements can also be used for reflection, allowing the clients to engage with previous creations.

Furthermore, cloud storage options such as Google Drive may be adopted as a space to document and keep a client's work, observing and returning to it in the future. The shared cloud storage can provide a group space for collaborative work, artistic responses, and dialogue between meetings, as long as privacy compliance rules are observed. Using Google Drive during pandemic lockdowns was very supportive for a group of elderly clients I worked with. It helped them to keep in contact, process complex feelings, and decrease loneliness in times where physical encounters were not possible.

Creation and Performance

The largest obstacles of virtual art therapy relate to finding ways of conducting artistic and performative work through the screen. Keeping a playful, experimental, and creative approach provides clients with ideas and inspiration for their own creative journey. My suggestion is to be spontaneous and use the screen as a stage. When facilitating movement or dramatic work, the therapist can use online features to inspire the clients by modeling in tandem with them. In addition, the therapist can use the spotlight feature in Zoom to highlight one participant. This feature automatically enlarges the camera feed of the spot lit individual, thereby providing a theatrical atmosphere for the presenter and audience.

Relating to the "shifting role" model (Berger, 2017, 2021), the therapist can shift between multiple roles:

- The actor (or artist, dancer, or musician): playing and creating for or with the clients
- The director or choreographer: giving instructions to explore and develop issues artistically
- The audience: witnessing and containing the work
- The producer: taking care of the setting and basic needs of members

Artistic presentations and performances can be improvised in the present moment. Alternatively, they can be created and rehearsed earlier, and then performed at a later date. They can be recorded and edited as video clips to be shown and shared with the therapist and group members during sessions, hence carrying the concept of "performance-based therapy" (Berger, 2021) into the virtual realm.

The Screen as a Stage

When working with individuals or smaller teams as part of a larger group, I often use the breakout room function in Zoom to allow for a meaningful group experience. Breakout rooms are a virtual splitting of a videoconferencing session in which participants are redirected to separate spaces from the main session. The Host can assign participants to specific rooms, thus maintaining some control over group dynamics. I typically begin with activities in a large group as a warm-up for participants and to set an example for the coming smaller groupwork. Providing the option of engaging in small groups through the use of breakout rooms allows participants that feel shy or embarrassed to have a more intimate and safe space for expression.

With some of my groups, the following framework became our weekly mode of working from session to session. The format stays the same while the stories and artistic responses change. The first phase begins in the large group when each participant is invited to create an artistic product in visual art, dance, music, writing, or drama. When they finish, they may share their creation with the group by showing it to the camera and, if they feel comfortable, providing commentary or writing the creation's title in the chat. Another option is to present the creations on a collective digital notice board, such as Padlet, where they have the same options of giving their work a title or writing a short sentence.

The second phase can be conducted in the large group as a demonstration, or directly in small groups. Following the therapist's explanation, participants are chosen for different roles: one as a presenter and four or five as artistic responders. The presenter shares their artwork, poem, or performance and has the opportunity to say a few words about their piece. Then a cycle of artistic responses begins, in which other participants echo the work back, using art forms to express the ways it touched them. Responses are given through music, art, poetry, and movement, or through a symbolic personal object that echoes the story back to the presenter. The echoes can be made one after the other with the non-presenting participants (the audience) turning off their camera to remain within the metaphoric artistic mode or by using the spotlight feature to highlight the responder. Alternatively, the echoing can be presented simultaneously using the screen as a collective stage for an interdisciplinary performance.

If time allows, this format can be used in breakout rooms, shifting the roles between participants. If time is sparse, only one or two participants can be invited to share, while the rest can be invited just to show their work or their titles. It is important to remember to conduct some kind of closure or farewell ritual in the breakout rooms before returning to the large group's collective ending.

Michelle Winkel shares her experience as the 'performer' in the demonstration phase at one of Ronen's large group sessions:

> I was initially hesitant to volunteer to step into the performer role because the group was very large, and I think of myself as a visual artist, not a performer. My comfort zone is quietly making art. However, Ronen prepared us for this particular group activity by raising the energy and awareness in playful and unexpected ways—for example, inviting us to dance, to mimic his body movements or choose our own, and to interpret the loud rap music coming through the computer audio from his studio to ours.
>
> He coached us out of our comfortable chairs. "Come on," he said. "Take space in your room, grow big, and bigger, now push the walls, the room is too small for you! And now you are liquid, you are oil, find your groove, you are flowing. Now write your name with your nose!" Dancing with more than one hundred colleagues was invigorating for me and brought another dimension to my feelings about this group and about myself. We then shifted to drawing and writing. We scribbled down words in a sketchbook, creating some short stories individually, quickly, and lightly. The stories flowed unusually easily for me. We were invited to strike out any words we did not want to share with anyone and write

"blah blah blah" or gibberish instead. They became poems of sorts. Ronen continued, "Now you are going to read it aloud to yourself. What kind of an audience do you imagine you're speaking to? Where are you standing as you read it? What kind of music do you hear?"

Moving to the playback theatre aspect of the workshop, I volunteered, along with five or six others, to perform while the large group watched with their cameras off. Suddenly, over 90 Zoom squares of faces went black, and while I knew they were still listening, it created a mood of privacy that seemed surreal to me. I was now alone with a small visible audience, and had a supportive facilitator in Ronen. He instructed the other volunteers to listen actively to my playback theatre—a dramatic reading of my poem, twice, in different styles. He prepared each of them to resonate with my enactment by making a response piece, conveying how my performance touched them. One responded through making a visual art response, one in movement, one through music, and one by a narrative. Then I stepped onto the Zoom stage. I performed my piece once, with anger rising in my voice and body, yelling, and all embarrassment left me. It was liberating. The anger shifted quickly. As I moved into the second reading of the poem, I suddenly felt sad, and yet very peaceful. I felt profoundly recognized as the others fed back their responses on the virtual stage, one by one.

This intermodal method works well for groups using the screen as a stage while incorporating the technology and its tools. It creates a group and communal experience and allows participants various ways of expression. Moving and shifting between roles and artistic styles expands creativity and flexibility, which are important coping mechanisms in a changing world (Berger, 2021).

Epilogue

This chapter presents concepts and methods to improve virtual arts-based work with groups. As the screen becomes a space for art making and a stage for artistic presentations, this chapter acknowledges the unique characteristics and meanings of the virtual spaces. Telecommunication platforms, such as Zoom, lend themselves for synchronous therapy use, while shared cloud servers, such as Google Drive, may set the stage for asynchronous art collaboration. Delivering arts-based therapy online, however, creates new dilemmas around participant relationships and ethical considerations. Examples from practice are used to highlight the implementation of methods with various clients and present the potential of these methods in the use of virtual art therapy in a changing world.

Concluding this chapter, my hope is that as more practitioners use and research virtual arts-based therapy, so, too, will the practice grow and improve. This process will allow more people to use art therapy, improving its accessibility to populations that have previously had difficulty connecting with a therapist in person.

References

Berger, R. (2017). Shifting roles: A new art-based creative supervision model. *The Arts in Psychotherapy, 55*, 158–163.

Berger, R. (2021). Shifting Roles: An Arts-Based Supervision Model. In R. Berger, *Arts Therapy in a Changing World* (pp. 175–199). New York: Nova.

Berger, R., & Liber, D. (2021). Beyond the Screen: Concepts, Methods, and Ethical Guidelines to Improve Arts-Based Therapy via Zoom. In R. Berger, *Arts Therapy in a Changing World* (pp. 269–295). New York: Nova.

Collie, K., & Čubranić, D. (1999). An art therapy solution to a telehealth problem. *Art Therapy: The Journal of the American Art Therapy Association, 16*(4), 186–193.

Pendzik, S. (1994). The theatre stage and sacred space. *The Arts in Psychotherapy, 21* (1), 25–35.

Shuper-Engelhard, E., & Furlager, A. Y. (2020). Remaining held: dance/movement therapy with children during lockdown. *Body, Movement and Dance in Psychotherapy*, 1–14.

8 Keeping Up With the Times

Art Therapy Moves from Studio to Chat Room to Zoom

Sara Prins Hankinson and Kate Collie

Introduction

Canada has a relatively small population spread across a vast geographical area with many people living in remote, rural, or northern communities where there is limited access to specialty health services. Telecommunications technologies, such as telephones and radios, have been used to facilitate telehealth—i.e., healthcare from a distance—in Canada for many decades (Cervinkas, 1984). When the internet emerged in the early 1990s, Canada became a telehealth leader and has since used the internet to make specialty care, including art therapy, more widely accessible.

As part of her work as an art therapist in a cancer centre, Prins Hankinson would plan support groups for families with counselors in other cities and, initially, drive to lead these groups in person. In 2013, she hosted a group for young adults with cancer using telehealth technology: they attended the group in person at a cancer centre that was an hour's drive away from her, and she relied on a counsellor there to set up the art supplies and connect to everyone by video. Later, she hosted annual four-week group sessions for young adult cancer patients using Skype for Business. In 2012, she connected with Kate Collie, who had been working on distance art therapy since 1998, and together, they developed CancerChatCanada (later: Cancer Chat). Their collaboration culminates in the virtual art therapy groups Prins Hankinson hosted in 2020 in response to COVID-19. In the discussion of the programs, this chapter presents the structure of the group sessions as well as client responses.

Online Art Therapy Groups for Cancer Care in Canada

In 2012, both Sara Prins Hankinson and Kate Collie worked at Canadian cancer centres: Sara in Vancouver, British Columbia, and Kate in Edmonton, Alberta. They began meeting and exploring what distance art therapy groups for cancer patients could look like with technology that was available then. They formed a team of art therapists in Canada and the US with a common interest in digital art therapy, and trialled online art making tools, apps, and

DOI: 10.4324/9781003149538-10

sessions held using Skype and Google Hangouts. Sara and Kate took turns leading mock art therapy groups with the rest of the team (Prins Hankinson et al., 2016).

They spent the majority of their time developing methods of hosting art therapy groups using CancerChatCanada. Evaluations of this pan-Canadian service were showing favorable results (Stephen et al., 2013, 2014) and Kate knew there was interest in expanding the program to include art therapy. The purpose of CancerChatCanada was, and still is under its new name of Cancer Chat at DeSouza Institute, to provide free and professionally led online support groups to Canadians affected by cancer, including patients, survivors, and family members. Sessions are typed (text-based, no voice/audio) and take place in real time, with all participants logging in at the same time to take part in the discussion. Groups meet once a week for 90 minutes, for 8 to 12 weeks, in a live online chat room. In 2013, Sara began hosting art therapy groups for patients on CancerChatCanada—first with a young adult population, and later opening it up to patients of any age.

In 2020, Cancer Chat still retained its low-tech accessibility, with just a chat room and a page for participants to post their artwork each week. However, the framework it provided proved valuable with the restrictions due to the COVID-19 pandemic. All in-person support services at the Cancer Centre were suspended, and Sara, like most others, was forced to figure out how to adapt. What follows is her description of what she did.

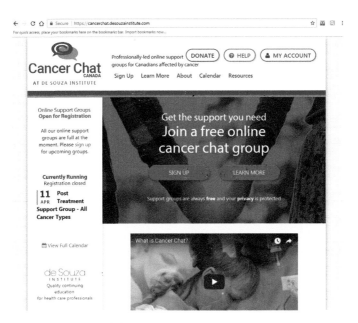

Figure 8.1 CancerChat's Website

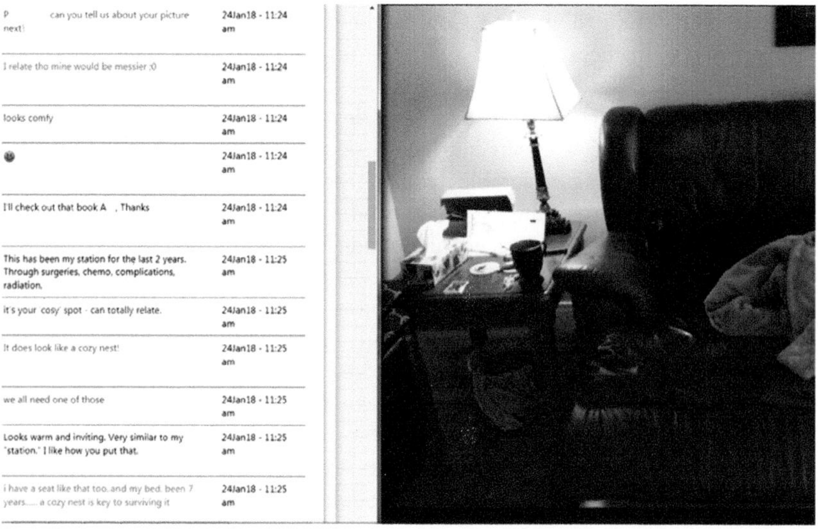

P can you tell us about your picture next!	24Jan18 - 11:24 am
I relate tho mine would be messier ;0	24Jan18 - 11:24 am
looks comfy	24Jan18 - 11:24 am
●	24Jan18 - 11:24 am
I'll check out that book A , Thanks	24Jan18 - 11:24 am
This has been my station for the last 2 years. Through surgeries, chemo, complications, radiation.	24Jan18 - 11:25 am
it's your cosy spot - can totally relate.	24Jan18 - 11:25 am
It does look like a cozy nest!	24Jan18 - 11:25 am
we all need one of those	24Jan18 - 11:25 am
Looks warm and inviting. Very similar to my 'station.' I like how you put that.	24Jan18 - 11:25 am
i have a seat like that too. and my bed. been 7 years..... a cozy nest is key to surviving it	24Jan18 - 11:25 am

Figure 8.2 CancerChatCanada Discussion of the Photograph of a Member's "Station"

Sara's Virtual Art Therapy Groups in 2020

I began the lockdown in the spring of 2020 by hosting a group on Cancer Chat for patients across Canada, as this was an easy first step for offering support to patients from a distance. In April, my workplace granted access to Zoom for Healthcare (a more secure version of Zoom) and I began to transition my in-person support groups to take place over Zoom, too. In our original CancerChatCanada groups, we had developed three models of chatting and creating art together: asynchronous, synchronous, and our mixed method (the group chat would be live (synchronous) and the art making would be done on their own time (asynchronous)). Our sessions were weekly and 90 minutes long.

In April 2020, I rolled out my first Zoom art therapy group with a small group of patients who were well connected from regularly attending an in-person art studio group. I knew they would be excited to see each other again and would give me feedback on these initial online art therapy experiences. After a few weeks, I felt more confident about hosting more groups using Zoom, and I started a second art therapy group open to all patients and caregivers across the province. There were four participants that initially signed up for the second group.

Knowing the great weight that group members would be carrying when experiencing cancer and the added restrictions and anxieties due to the pandemic, I titled the second group *Art for Self Care*. The format that I typically followed for each session is shown in Table 8.1.

These first two groups became very close and looked forward to the weekly sessions as this was one of the few social functions and support services available to most of them during that time. Over the summer, I changed the

Table 8.1 Weekly Format of "Art for Self Care" Group

Time	Activity
1:30–1:45	Going around the "circle" to see how everyone was doing that week
1:45–2:00	Sharing resources—allowing them space to share anything they found helpful
2:00–2:30	Reviewing the artwork made by participants each week in a Power-Point presentation
2:30–2:40	A guided meditation or visualization
2:40–2:55	A simple drawing exercise they could do beside their computer with just a pen and paper
2:55–3:00	Offering the group an optional "creative challenge" or art homework for them to complete during the week

group to take place bi-weekly and the participants provided feedback that they missed the weekly event. For the fall of 2020, I chose monthly themed groups to invite more participants, with group members signing up to attend one month at a time. Table 8.2 shows the themes of the monthly groups.

In addition, I co-hosted a monthly music and art therapy group with a music therapist using the same format. However, we designed this group as a four-week program where participants discovered a different fine art modality and music therapy experience each session. We incorporated live music, songs streamed from YouTube, and connected to other apps in this group.

Interest grew, and while in the spring these groups mostly contained 3–5 people, in the fall of 2020 they had 10–13 participants. There was more time spent checking in on everyone and looking at their artwork from week to week, and less time spent sharing resources and being led in a guided meditation (aside from the Mindfulness-Based Art Therapy group.)

Knowing about the challenge of "Zoom fatigue" (Lee, 2020) and wanting to keep these groups a comfortable and creative space, I found it was valuable to shift between viewing all of the participants together on the screen and turning our attention to a shared screen, such as for viewing the artwork together. Before each session, participants emailed me a photo of something they had made if they felt comfortable sharing it with the group. I then compiled the artwork into a PowerPoint presentation to share. This was a valuable way of honoring the artwork, as we all looked closely at what was created. It also

Table 8.2 Themes of Monthly Art Therapy Groups

Month	Theme
September	Art Therapy 101
October	Photographing the Fall
November	Mindfulness-Based Art Therapy
December	Wrapping Up the Year (creative reflections to close 2020)

provided the space for each participant to share more naturally in a video-conferencing setting.

The Whiteboard function on Zoom is a tool that I used regularly to lead the group in a drawing exercise. With it, they can see me drawing mandalas, Zentangles, spirals, and other forms of meditative doodling and can draw along with me.

I also regularly implemented resources from the internet into our sessions. I played audio meditations found online and we watched short videos from YouTube together. There was one session when we even went on a virtual trip to an art gallery together to view a Picasso exhibit. We reviewed online resource pages for cancer patients, showed art ideas, and showed inspirational webpages as part of our session.

Benefits of Zoom Art Therapy Groups

I missed rolling out the tablecloths and setting up a table with art materials that patients eagerly dive into (or hesitantly try if it is their first time and they are overwhelmed with possibility). I missed the small conversations that happen organically at each end of the table which can't quite happen within a Zoom group. I missed having control over the therapeutic environment—knowing that each participant is safe and has the appropriate art supplies to participate in the activities.

However, there have been many advantages to hosting art therapy groups using Zoom for healthcare—some expected, some unexpected. First, there is the advantage of having an online space available to host groups whenever I would like it. When working within a hospital, finding an available conference room to turn into a temporary art studio was a challenge—first, finding a time that it was available, and then hauling the art supplies from a closet on the top floor down to the conference room, and back again. With Zoom, I can host a group whenever I would like. Additionally, I don't have to set up and clean up art supplies. This is a time savings of about an hour per group session.

Coming into the hospital for an art therapy session was a barrier for many patients. While my mandate is to provide support for patients throughout the province, I had never seen anyone from the North or the Interior in my groups, nor had I been able to travel to those places. For the first time, people in these regions began accessing art therapy services on Zoom. Furthermore, patients located in urban centres that could access in-person support services sometimes chose not to because entering the hospital again brought back traumatizing memories.

From April to October 2020, 40 patients participated in Zoom art therapy groups. They were given a link to fill out an online survey regarding their experience of the group. Below is a summary of the benefits mentioned on the 18 surveys that were returned. Most were in response to the question "What did you find to be the most helpful part of the distance art therapy group?"

Accessibility

As mentioned above, accessibility was a major advantage to hosting the group virtually. One person wrote that the most helpful part was "connecting with others without traveling 25 minutes by car each way to class." Others mentioned the savings in parking fees.

Having participants attend from around the province proved to be an enriching experience. We learned about their home and saw how varied the landscape and climate could be. One person wrote: "I found that hearing about what was happening in their part of [the province] made me feel less confined as I was not leaving my home because of the COVID situation."

Comfortability of Attending from Home

There is an ease in attending groups from home—I felt it in wearing my slippers, sipping a cup of coffee from my favorite mug while I worked. Everyone is in their own comfortable territory instead of stepping into a place where they are a visitor. Participants have said they feel more at ease, and some have even attended while laying on their couch or in their bed. Zoom can prove to be an inviting space for someone who is shy, as they can choose their level of participation. One person reported, "I would have found a real roomful of strangers inhibiting, whereas on Zoom I could hold back and participate to the degree I was comfortable."

Connection

Participants reported feeling a real sense of fellowship within the group and appreciated the opportunity to connect with other cancer patients. It created a sense of belonging, and it was a safe space to explore feelings, art, experiment, relate, and create friendships. This experience was especially important during this time of the pandemic, when most participants were rarely leaving their homes and felt isolated.

Emotional Support

Most participants were undergoing chemotherapy, radiation treatments, or both during the time of this group. Some of them had surgeries scheduled and all of them had regular scans and appointments—all anxiety provoking. With COVID-19, their appointments and support networks were upended, anxiety increased, and there were fewer people with whom to connect. Patients reported that "the sessions helped me get through a tough emotional time." The group and art therapy exercises "[gave] me some ways to deal with the shock and anxiety of my cancer experience."

Weekly Structure

There were only a few participants of the Zoom art therapy groups that were working – the rest were retired or on medical leave. Several of them lived alone and had few commitments. Being immunocompromised, most of them seldom ventured into public spaces aside from appointments. The weekly art therapy sessions became one of their few regular commitments. Several people said that they spent significant time each week thinking about each session, and that they looked forward to every session. For instance, one artist discovered that she enjoyed working with chalk pastels in this drawing of her summer cabin (Figure 8.3), where she wished she could be.

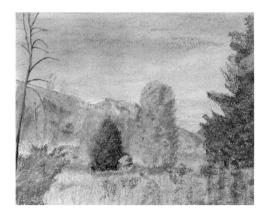

Figure 8.3 A Group Participant's Drawing of Where She Would Like to Be

Homework Inspiration

In not being able to attend an art studio that was set up for them, patients had to make their own creative space and set aside time for homework. I believe this made them more involved in their therapeutic process and gave them more incentive to develop their creative process. Several people wrote about the value of these "homework assignments." The art therapy projects provided inspiration and they delighted in what they were able to learn and create from week to week, and in seeing how others took the same assignment and came up with something different. Figure 8.4 on the following page shows an example of a woman who discovered that she enjoyed drawing.

Connection Beyond the Zoom Art Therapy Sessions

Participants reported finding friends within the Zoom art therapy group, and some began keeping in touch with each other outside of the group sessions. Moreover, participants reported connecting more with others outside of the group. One woman wrote,

I started taking photos of flowers and other things in my garden as a basis for our homework projects, and found myself sharing my photos with friends on email and strengthening my social connections with old friends while isolated by the COVID situation.

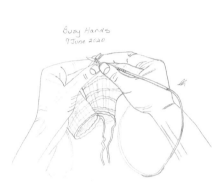

Figure 8.4 Drawing by a Woman who "Discovered I Could Draw and That I Really Enjoy Drawing"

There were a couple of people who reported feeling connected to the group even when they weren't able to attend because of the weekly email that was sent. This contained a link to the next meeting as well as a recap of the session and the "creative challenge."

Challenges of Zoom Art Therapy Groups

The transition to online was more difficult with the young adults' group. Before the pandemic, the group regularly saw approximately ten well-connected patients show up and leave to grab coffee together afterwards. Only four chose to keep attending the group when the transition was made to an online format. One person wrote that, although distance art therapy is better than nothing, "in person is always better."

Furthermore, I was not able to determine a way to facilitate the children's group to take place via Zoom. I previously hosted this group with a nurse and a counselor. We led several families through the experience of art activities, snacking, educational lessons on cancer, and round-table sharing. The best alternative I came up with was individual family art therapy sessions on Zoom, where I read the kids a story and we did art activities together with some supplies that I had mailed to them.

There are also limitations when it comes to what art therapy activities can be offered to clients. I can mail some supplies to participants, but this is bound to what can fit in an envelope or package, so options are limited. Most of the art activities have been adapted so that they can be simple drawing or photography exercises, or done with whatever materials patients already have on hand.

Another challenge were the distractions that occurred during our Zoom art therapy sessions. Children sometimes made appearances on the screen, and one woman was mortified when her landlord knocked on her door to collect a late rental payment during our group session. Some seemed more comfortable making trips to the washroom and fridge during our time together than others. These things were all out of our control as group participants, and sometimes we sat in some awkwardness as we witnessed what was going on in another's environment. The best we could do was mute or unmute microphones and continue to try to make everyone feel comfortable in the online space.

Sometimes there were technical issues, although I have been impressed with how little this has happened with Zoom. Most people adapted quickly. Some, however, admitted to not really knowing how to use Zoom except getting into and out of the session. There were times where we worked with the group member experiencing difficulties and came up with a solution together. It was a bonding experience with other group members suggesting solutions from their experience—we were all figuring this thing out together. Some said that they didn't mind their limited knowledge of Zoom; when offered the opportunity to use the chat box and other features, they declined.

There was also one critique on sharing artwork. One person wrote that it was not what she had anticipated, but she did it because she felt comfortable in the small group setting. Guidelines are now given at the beginning of the group to let people know that they can choose between keeping their art to themselves, sharing with just the art therapist, or sharing with the group.

Opportunities for Development

There is the potential to incorporate digital mediums into Zoom art therapy sessions. Screens from tablets can be shared within a Zoom session. This could allow for the facilitator to share what they are drawing on their iPad, or participants to be able to share what they are working on with their device. In the music and art therapy group I co-led, the music therapist was able to link in her iPad, which has a spectrograph app on it. With the app on our shared screen in the session, she was able to record participants' voices and take a screenshot of the sound waves their voices made. Participants then created images inspired by the picture of what their voice looked like. A session like this was only possible because of the ability Zoom provided to link devices.

Photography also worked well within the context of a Zoom art therapy session. Perhaps future sessions could include video storytelling, with participants creating their own videos using online software. Zoom is an ideal platform for watching videos together. Similarly, websites and apps with art-making capacity could be easily shown and shared within a session.

Conclusion

Earlier experiences in distance art therapy using CancerChatCanada and other digital mediums laid the groundwork for Zoom art therapy groups to take place during the pandemic of 2020. Despite the challenges, patients appreciated the opportunity to access this support service—some of them for the first time.

The weekly Zoom art therapy sessions provided clients with structure, emotional support regarding anxiety, community during a time of isolation, and inspiration through cancer treatments and post-treatment recovery. Because patients had to create their own space for art therapy, they became more active in their therapeutic process. Many seemed to have invested in art supplies with the money they would have spent on parking. They created an art therapy space in their home and found new confidence in their creativity and connection with group members from afar.

For decades, we dipped our toes into distance art therapy and then were thrust into it in 2020. Now that we are in this space and we have discovered the advantages of distance art therapy, we believe that we are here to stay.

References

Cervinkas, J. (1984). *Telehealth: Telecommunications technology in health care and health education in Canada*. Canadian Commission for UNESCO.

Lee, J. (2020). A Neurological Exploration of Zoom Fatigue. *Psychiatric Times*. https://www.psychiatrictimes.com/view/psychological-exploration-zoom-fatigue.

Prins Hankinson, S., Jones, B., & Collie, K. (2016). Adapting Art Therapy for Online Groups. In E. Horovitz & S. Brooke (Eds.) *Combining the creative therapies with technology: Using social media and online counseling to treat clients* (pp. 34–52). Charles Thomas, Springfield IL USA.

Stephen, J., Rojubally, A., MacGregor, K., McLeod, D., Speca, M., Taylor-Brown, J., Fergus, K., Collie, K., Turner, J., Sellick, S., & MacKenzie, G. (2013). Evaluation of CancerChatCanada: A program of online support for Canadians affected by cancer. *Current Oncology, 20*(1), 39–47.

Stephen, S., Collie, K., McLeod, D., Rojubally, A., Fergus, K., Speca, M., Turner, J., Taylor-Brown, J., Sellick, S., Burrus, K., & Elramly, M. (2014). Talking with Text: Therapeutic Communication in CancerChatCanada Support Groups. *Social Science & Medicine 104*, 178–186. doi:10.1016/j.socscimed.2013.12.001.

9 Reaching Older Adults Through Virtual Art Therapy

Margaret Carlock-Russo

Introduction

Older adults are often faced with many losses as they age. Some of these include family, home, identity, purpose, partnership, and sometimes even memories. Art therapy can be an effective support for navigating daily life and a means to maintain cognitive stimulation, social connections, a sense of purpose, self-worth, and preserve personal identity for individuals with advancing memory loss and other medical issues (Guseva, 2019) as well as provide stress relief and support to their caregivers (Hunt et al., 2018). For years, I have practiced art therapy with many individuals struggling to maintain these qualities in their own lives, regardless of their ages. In early 2016, I was hired to create an art therapy program for this purpose in a "Life Plan" Community in Southern Arizona. This type of community is designed for individuals and couples ages 55 and older who are living independently when they move into the community. In addition, there is a care centre in the community for any resident who develops an illness or condition that requires assistance with daily living or skilled nursing care. I was employed to develop an art therapy program within the care centre, particularly focusing on services for those living with dementia.

This chapter explores the change in my art therapy approach as I transitioned from in-person sessions to online with a population that needed extra support to deal with the added technological as well as therapeutic challenges.

What Causes Dementia?

Dementia is a general term for a decline in mental ability severe enough to interfere with daily life (Alzheimer's Association, 2020). There are many different types of illnesses and conditions that cause dementia. Dementia is a general term describing a wide range of symptoms associated with declining cognitive skills, including memory, that are severe enough to impede a person's ability to perform everyday activities (American Psychological Association, 2013). There are many conditions that can cause dementia, including vascular, Lewy body, and frontotemporal dementia, in addition to Alzheimer's Disease, which is the most

DOI: 10.4324/9781003149538-11

common type of dementia and accounts for 60 to 80 percent of dementia cases (Alzheimer's Association, 2020). Ultimately, dementia is caused by damaged brain cells. The damage interferes with the ability of brain cells to communicate with each other. When brain cells cannot communicate normally, thinking, behaviour, and feelings can be affected (Alzheimer's Association, 2020).

Symptoms of dementia can vary greatly, and caution must be taken when assessing dementia in an individual since other medical conditions can cause dementia-like symptoms, such as depression, reactions to medications, and endocrine abnormalities. Although it is common in older individuals, dementia is not a normal part of the ageing process. Younger individuals can exhibit signs of dementia as well (Alzheimer's Association, 2020). At least two of the following core mental functions must be significantly impaired to be diagnosed (American Psychological Association, 2013):

- Memory
- Communication and language
- Ability to focus
- Reasoning and judgement
- Visual perception

Our life experiences create neural patterns in signal type and strength. These patterns explain how, at the cellular level, our brains code our thoughts, memories, skills, and sense of who we are. As we meet new people, have new experiences, and acquire new skills, activity patterns change. Patterns also change when Alzheimer's disease or a related disorder disrupts nerve cells and their connections to one another (National Institute on Aging, 2017). Engaging in creative arts activities in community can help a person with dementia maintain a sense of belonging, express themselves non-verbally, organize their thoughts, and cope with a variety of changes and challenges they may be facing (Betts, 2018).

Developing a Community Art Therapy Program

As I developed the art therapy program in 2016, a few realities quickly became apparent: I needed to educate potential participants about what art therapy is, how I practice, and what benefits might be derived from participation—not only for the individual with dementia, but also for loved ones, caregivers, and staff involved in that person's life. I engaged in a process of providing basic information about art therapy as well as types of dementia along with experiential opportunities. I took the approach of involving everyone, not just the individuals living with cognitive decline.

Because the initial goal was more focused on getting people involved, I used an art as therapy, strengths-based approach and encouraged interactions among participants. This accomplished two important things: first, it created a cohesive community without singling any particular group out. Secondly, it allowed staff and family members to see the participants with dementia from a different lens. The focus was on capabilities rather than limitations. Verbal interactions, while present, were not the main way of engaging and communicating among group members. While it took some time for folks to become involved, once they did, it was easier for them to understand the potential benefits.

This kind of approach allowed participants to gain experience and education over time in a manner that was easier to absorb because they were also seeing real-time examples of the potential benefits for their loved ones. They learned about the struggles that manifest for those with dementia and how to identify behaviours that might indicate that a person is feeling challenged, confused, or overwhelmed. Additionally, caregivers began to experience some benefits of their own, such as relaxation, stress relief, and being able to engage in an enjoyable activity with their loved one. Staff began to understand the non-pharmacological benefits of art therapy and were open to encouraging participation opportunities, especially for individuals exhibiting anxiousness, exit-seeking behaviours, or confusion. Over time, everyone involved learned that participating in art therapy group sessions often contributed to a more productive and pleasant day for all involved.

Some of the difficulties that a person with a dementia-causing condition may experience are listed in Table 9.1 along with potential coping behaviours they may exhibit in response to the stressors they experience.

When meeting in-person, it was possible to identify and navigate the observable clues that participants were sharing. I could use the personal familiarity and relationship-based therapeutic approaches to address some of the concerns as well as redirect and distract someone from the adverse environmental triggers they were experiencing. I became a living cue and connection to the art therapy group by association. Facilitating groups in person allowed me great flexibility in how I motivated and encouraged participation, arranged the environment, introduced media and materials, engaged assistance, and arranged transportation to groups.

Practicing in a New Environment

At the end of February 2020, after establishing and providing the art therapy program for four years, I had the opportunity to move on to some other projects,

Table 9.1 How Brain Changes Impact a Person

Difficulty Exhibited	Coping Behaviour
Expressing self	Withdrawal/less verbal engagement
Making choices	Avoiding interactions
Following directions	Anxiousness
Feeling safe/secure	Clinging behaviour
Recognizing people	Repetitive questions
Slower processing of information	Inability to answer questions

so I reallocated the community program to another art therapist. Within two weeks, the United States announced the COVID pandemic, and everything changed. I couldn't create new groups as I had hoped so I regrouped and pivoted my plans to move toward an online model. Naively, I thought it would be easy to locate interested caregivers to participate. In those first few months of pandemic restrictions, I tried reaching out through social media, local support groups, and organizations. It seemed as though everything was on hold. Although I began to offer online groups, it was difficult to offer specific groups for older adults, caregivers, or individuals with dementia.

I needed to rethink the approach I used in-person to be successful online. I had to learn more about virtual platforms, reconsider accessibility, adjust media, and figure out strategies to promote engagement while not exacerbating confusion or losing attention too quickly. I attended several online art therapy trainings through the American Art Therapy Association and the Canadian Art Therapy Association that were very helpful. Some issues were addressed in the teletherapy training I attended and by discussing options with colleagues. Others were sorted out through trial and error.

In those initial groups, I navigated participants' technological challenges in locating the meeting link and logging in correctly. For example, one older woman consistently required reminding and assistance in positioning her screen so she would be visible during the session. A participant in a unique group that I offered for caregivers and their loved ones (LO) with cognitive decline spent almost half of the first group session just trying to connect to the virtual platform. While technical difficulties may happen occasionally, I was concerned that the pressure and overwhelm of the more complicated access would affect participants adversely. I discovered quickly that including caregivers as partners in online sessions proved essential to the successful engagement of older adult participants. There were some people who refused to register, despite their caregiver's encouragement, because of the potential challenges and discomfort when meeting virtually. In hindsight, it was probably better that I began with a few small groups. It allowed me to quickly correct things that weren't serving the group and develop a structure that worked for the participants.

For individuals who were already dealing with challenges understanding their environments, the sudden changes and increased isolation required to quell the spread of the COVID-19 virus wreaked their own havoc. For people living with dementia, sudden changes in daily life, such as moving to a new setting, deaths of loved ones, loss of skills, memory recall, and loss of identity and purpose in life can produce confusion, anxiety, and isolation that may be difficult to manage. One of the most important things you can do for a person with dementia is to keep their daily routine as consistent as possible. Engaging in meaningful activities can help a person feel safe and secure and also provide a sense of purpose. I mention purpose often because I find it to be one of the most central needs for people I work with. These are all individuals who led successful lives, had families, jobs, and community activities, and now they had nothing to replace those parts of their lives. Taking a person-centred (Thorne & Sanders, 2013) positive approach to focus on a person's abilities rather than their deficits promotes a strength-based and success-oriented therapy. Below are the basic principles I follow when using this approach.

Intervention focuses on the person-centred, strengths-based approach:

- Dignity, social engagement, communication, relaxation
- Processing of life transitions/diagnoses
- End-of-life care
- Non-pharmacological approaches to care
- Focus on individual strengths
- Empowerment/agency

When I develop interventions for in-person sessions, it is almost always with input from the client, either verbally or non-verbally. I strive to promote the understanding that we are a team, and I am there to support them. In this way, I can put the client at ease, and they often are more willing to engage, especially if they feel that they are contributing in some way. In all interactions, I focus on sustaining dignity, social engagement, and sense of purpose. I try to relate the interventions to areas of the client's life when they felt most capable and contributed to society. I let the client lead me and I meet them where they are.

Originally, I expected working in a virtual model to be vastly similar to the in-person model I created. While my person-centred style and overall goals of providing a sense of purpose, validation, self-expression, and social interaction remained, I discovered that I had to alter many aspects of my approach. I became acutely aware of how much I relied on non-verbal cues and personal interactions to foster rapport and promote group cohesion in person. There was, however, much less visibility in a virtual model. We were unable to see each other's mannerisms or non-verbal cues and observing the creation of an image was difficult. I could no longer sit next to someone and model how to hold a brush, utilize a particular media, or provide an adaptive tool. I had to rely much more on verbal interactions. Particularly with people experiencing confusion and environmental awareness issues, verbal instruction and communication brought its own set of complications. Multi-step and long verbal exchanges could actually diminish receptivity and involvement rather than promote it.

To maintain comfortable exchanges and minimize confusion, I decided to send emails to participants in advance of group sessions. In the emails, I provided some background about art therapy and my approach. This information took the place of some of the initial education I tended to do with in-person groups. I included the theme, a suggested materials list, and any other helpful information so the caregivers could prepare items and familiarize themselves with the process in advance of the group meeting.

Group members with cognitive decline also received the emails so they can be aware of what to expect. Sometimes those messages needed to be read aloud or be reviewed several times to increase understanding. Emails reduced the need for extensive directions or explanations in the group and allowed participants to engage with the media and materials more readily. Once involved in image making, most participants were able to focus on creating independently after materials had been set up. Caregivers engaged in the process alongside their LO. My increased reliance on caregivers was very different than with in-person groups. While it may seem that more burden was being put on the caregivers, I believe that they were also learning ways to engage with their LO and, hopefully, will be able to use some of the engagement techniques in their own interactions with their LO.

During one session, a participant became deeply engaged in creating with watercolour crayons which allowed the caregiver to focus on their own image more fully. During sharing and processing of the images, the caregiver shared how meaningful it was for her to be able to create together with her mother. Both mother and daughter shared their images and were able to acknowledge their feelings around being able to do something 'fun' together. I viewed this as an important connection point between the pair as well as an opportunity for the daughter to see the mother as an individual, recognizing her still-vital imagination and awareness.

It may seem unconventional to facilitate groups with both caregivers and older adults. Yet caregivers are essential to the success of a virtual model with people with cognitive and physical decline. They can ensure that technology is accessible, materials available, and often promote involvement from their LO. I can think of several occasions when, without another person troubleshooting technological mishaps, the group member with cognitive decline would have been unable to participate in the group. At one time or another, we have experienced everything from internet instability, microphone malfunction, meeting room link breaks, proper positioning of the camera, to moving of

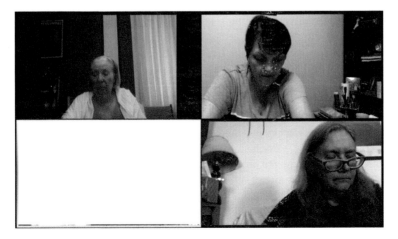

Figure 9.1 Group Session with Individuals Experiencing Cognitive Decline

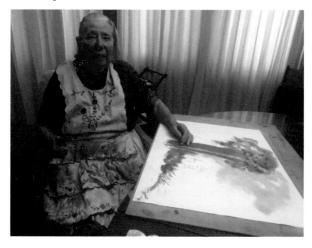

Figure 9.2 Group Member Sharing an Image She Created in an Online Group

computer equipment from one room to another. I can see how just one of those issues would have rendered the group member unable to join the group and perhaps lose interest.

One deficit of this model is that individuals may not feel as much privacy in the group, which could impact the level of disclosure in their processing. In my experience so far, this has not been an issue, although I continually monitor it. If there was a person who appeared to be uncomfortable sharing in the group, I would offer an opportunity to share individually at another time. Overwhelmingly, participants seemed to gain more than not, especially in spending enjoyable time together, sharing stories about their images, interacting socially, actively creating, and sharing ideas and opinions, which is often validating for the individual. For example, a group participant, called G, was able to share verbally about how she looked forward to these groups because they were the only times during the week that she interacted with others. G also expressed enjoyment about having her daughter participating with her. The presence of G's daughter actually seemed to enhance G's experience, as evidenced by her comment: "I am so excited for these groups each week. I don't know what I will do when they end." When I reassured her that we had several sessions left, she smiled and moved her arms as if cheering. Having opportunities to create visual images has also been helpful for G, a former teacher who enjoyed painting for many years. The physical process of using art media has encouraged not only reminiscence but also opportunities to share feelings of loss around physical changes. Through the sessions, G has been able to acknowledge some of the capabilities she does have and find ways to integrate them more fully, supporting her self-image.

Working virtually as a facilitator, I have to be much more flexible. One thing I rarely did when facilitating in-person sessions was to create images

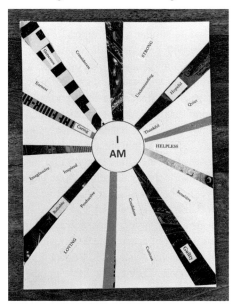

Figure 9.3 Sample "I am" Collage from a Group Image Prompt

alongside clients. While I acknowledge this process can be helpful with some clients, for the people I worked with, it sometimes distracted them. In addition, much of my time was spent moving from participant to participant providing support, cues, and redirection. Now I create my own imagery in every group. Because of the virtual format, I find it helps clients engage when they see me engaging. I also notice that when processing, they often expect me to share as well. I do tend to keep my images simple and my sharing basic and brief in order to keep the focus on the group. My sharing seems to positively affect the therapeutic relationship in my online groups. Changes take time, and I find learning happens together, often by trial and error. Most of my clients are understanding and flexible as we navigate this new experience together. It brings me back to my original instincts to work as partners from a person-centred frame. All participants have agency to make the group process better. This in itself can be a valuable therapeutic experience.

There are some unique benefits to online groups for this population. For instance, attendance is more consistent because transportation or even some minor health issues no longer pre-empt attendance. For clients who live at home and cannot travel, virtual art therapy makes connection with others and being part of a group a reality.

Early on, one of my concerns was that it would be difficult for participants to maintain attention to a relatively small screen. So far, this has not been an issue. The format of the session allows for greetings, brief introductions of themes, and then extended time creating, which helps mitigate screen fatigue.

The group closes with voluntary sharing of images, discussion, and a moment of gratitude. The format, while similar to an in-person group, is more predictable, which is helpful for those with cognitive difficulties.

Media has also changed. Previously, I often provided a selection of media for the group to choose from and suggested a theme or directive to focus the participants. In virtual groups, I suggest media for a particular theme while keeping options more flexible and open to whatever participants have on hand. I tend to identify common materials and items that can be easily found around the home. If a participant has access to more sophisticated or traditional art media, they are encouraged to incorporate what they like. I want to be sure that participants with limited access to media also feel included and able to engage.

Our biggest hurdle yet has been technology itself. I've learned that even with the best-laid plans, unexpected obstacles will pop up. We've had to deal with internet outages, storms that interrupted power service, and even time zone confusion. The groups have developed a level of acceptance and flexibility when members have challenges connecting. I think this has brought a new opportunity to foster support of one another among members. They empathize with others' situations.

The format that has been most successful with my participants is a one-hour session offered at the same time each week. I provide a link to access the group, which minimizes difficulty navigating online access. This provides consistency, routine, and predictability for participants. The one-hour duration is designed to allow sufficient time for engagement with media and processing without becoming too taxing or tiring for participants. I want group members to leave each session with a sense of accomplishment and connection that will inspire interest in attending future groups.

If anything has been validated through this experience, it is that people crave support and connection. There is a sense of belonging which is less about the way the group is facilitated and more about listening to members' needs and addressing those as best as possible. As we all have learned this last year, flexibility, patience, and creativity can help us reach our goals.

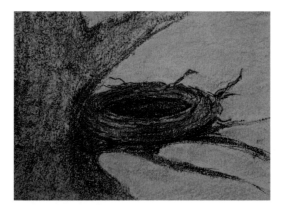

Figure 9.4 Personal Image Created in Group with a Prompt Focused on Nurturing

Session Ideas and Media

As I've mentioned previously, media can be difficult to manage given the online platform. There are situations where a facilitator or organization may be able to locally distribute media supplies to participants, which is a great asset. In this case, I decided to rely on common materials found in most living environments for two reasons: first, I wanted to be sure anyone with interest would be able to participate despite having limited access to traditional art media. Second, I wanted to demystify art making and use mostly familiar, recognizable elements so that participants could see this as a viable alternative for self-expression in the future. I focused each session using a few basic supplies with enough variations that most people would be able to access at least some of the listed items.

Collage was used in the beginning to reduce anxiety around artistic ability that may exist and to mitigate dexterity and organizational issues for any group members. Eventually, as group members gained confidence creating imagery, I incorporated a few more traditional materials for those that were interested. Even in doing so, the initial prompts encouraged freeform lines and shapes to minimize stress over the ability to render recognizable images. Three of the initial prompts are listed below. While I created these prompts, the ideas are not originally mine and are used widely in art therapy and expressive arts therapy. I credited sources where they were known.

(1) Prompt Title: Introductions (Collage)

Materials: (gathered at participant homes)

Blank paper—any size or type is fine
Something to use to trace a circle onto the paper (a bowl, paper plate, roll of masking tape, etc.)
Several clipped magazine or newspaper images
Additional colourful paper—old wrapping paper, printer paper, tissue paper, etc. (optional)
Glue stick or white glue
Writing or drawing implements, pens, pencils, markers, etc.

Process: Introduce collage process and use of circle shape to provide a boundary. Invite participants to create an image that reflects one or more things that bring joy to their lives.

(2) Prompt Title: I Am (Collage)

Materials: (words and phrases emailed by facilitator and other supplies gathered at participants home)

Facilitator emails a series of descriptive words and phrases to each participant to be printed out and used during the session. If printing is not possible, perhaps the list can be mailed. Participants can also cut out their own word options from newspapers, magazines, etc. (This may provide a secondary activity and a way to continue engagement when sessions are not scheduled.)

Blank paper, at least 8"x10" in size, with the words 'I AM' printed or written in the centre (copier/printer paper, cardboard, tag board, drawing paper, etc.)
Glue stick or white glue
Scissors (if appropriate), but paper can also be hand-torn and not cut
Several colourful collage paper strips, cut or torn from magazines or decorative papers
Writing and drawing implements (optional)

Process: Invite participants to engage in creating a collage using colourful magazine strips and descriptive words to form an image that represents their personality and way of being.

(3) Prompt Title: Emotions Study (adapted from a prompt shared by Nadia Paredes)

Materials: (this prompt can be utilized with a variety of media on paper)

Blank heavy gauge paper—as large as possible, up to 18"x24" (watercolour paper, card stock, tag board, etc.)
Drawing materials such as coloured pencils, pastels, markers, etc.
Watercolour pencils or paints, if available
Paintbrush and paint water cup, if available

Process: First, instruct participants, step-by-step, to fold their paper in half, and then in half again to create four quadrants on their paper. For visual clarity, lines can be drawn in the centre of the paper, one vertically and one horizontally, to create four sections on the paper. Begin by asking the participants to fill each section on the paper with lines and colour that reflect a particular emotion to them. Emotions are introduced one-by-one, with time to create before moving on to the next emotion. I used happy, angry, how you feel at this moment, and peaceful/ calm. You can use whatever feelings seem most appropriate for your group.

While these groups are relatively new, and more experience is necessary, early implications seem positive. Despite the learning curve and challenges that come with virtual art therapy, there are several benefits that make it likely to continue into the future. For people with dementia and their caregivers, online access often provides a more manageable avenue for participation, especially together, than traditional in-person models. The financial cost for transportation, additional caregivers, and travel supplies may also be reduced. Fatigue can be minimized as well. By limiting disruption of routine and time, the clients are able to use their energy to focus on the group experience without becoming overly tired or inattentive. My initial concerns about the viability of remote access have been largely debunked. The benefit of a participant with dementia and a caregiver being able to engage in a group together provides a unique opportunity to experience each other in a different context. This alone may promote greater understanding and intimacy for the pair.

Conclusion

The COVID-19 pandemic influenced the way art therapists worked with their clients. For older adults with advancing memory loss and other medical issues, navigating digital technology to participate in online art therapy sessions was often unrealistic and challenging at best. As I learned more about teletherapy and examined the essential components of what made my in-person art therapy sessions successful, I was able to create a group therapy model that allowed older adults experiencing physical and cognitive issues to successfully engage in online art therapy sessions. Including caregivers as partners and participants in the sessions created opportunities for both individuals to address personal, social, and emotional needs, as well as engage in new experiences together. While several adjustments were required to effectively facilitate partner groups virtually, it seems, at least in the groups I have facilitated, that the benefits outweigh the deficits. Clients in need of physical assistance setting up materials or navigating the virtual session space received that support from their caregiver partners and were able to engage in interventions to maintain cognitive stimulation, social connections, a sense of purpose, self-worth, and preserve personal identity while their caregiver partners learned new ways to interact with them as they participated in their own stress-relieving self-expression.

References

Alzheimer's Association. (2020). *What is Dementia?* Retrieved October 20, 2020 from https://www.alz.org/alzheimers-dementia/what-is-dementia.

American Psychological Association. (2013). *Diagnostic and statistical manual of mental disorders* (5th ed.). Washington, DC: APA.

Betts, D. (2018). Activating expression, connection, and transformation to enhance meaning and renew existence. *Art Therapy, 35*(3). 114–116. doi:10.1080/07421656.2018.1532690.

Guseva, E. (2019) Art therapy in dementia care: Toward neurologically informed, evidence-based practice. *Art Therapy, 36*(1), 46–49. doi:10.1080/07421656.2019.1564613.

Hunt, B., Truran, L., & Reynolds, F. (2018) "Like a drawing of breath": leisure-based art-making as a source of respite and identity among older women caring for loved ones with dementia. *Arts & Health, 10*(1), 29–44. doi:10.1080/17533015.2016.1247370.

National Institute on Aging. (2017). What happens to the brain in Alzheimer's Disease? Retrieved October 22, 2020 from https://www.nia.nih.gov/health/what-happens-brain-alzheimers-disease.

Thorne, B., & Sanders, P. (2013). *Carl Rogers*. 3rd edition. London: Sage.

Section 3

Innovations in Training and Supervision

10 Squaring The Schaverien Triangle

Lucille Proulx

Introduction

Supervision in art therapy is a relationship of learning. It provides opportunities for individuals less experienced in the field to reflect about their practicum work under the guidance of someone more experienced. For art therapists already in practice, supervision allows them to go deeper in understanding the spontaneous expressions in the artwork.

I began as a supervisor in 2001 in a face-to-face format, with the original artwork and the clients' reactions being discussed and examined. Later, I became associated with the Canadian International Institute of Art Therapy (CiiAT), which offers art therapy in a distance learning format. This also changed the delivery of supervision. Many of the art therapy students lived away from the city where the school was located and had to be supervised through internet and telephone communication.

I was concerned whether I would be able to work with the transference at a distance. It was surprising to see how well my first online student was able to describe the client session in emails and prepare for our telephone meeting. Over time, I became attuned to the vocabulary used to describe the sessions in the email, and when discussing the artwork by telephone, the tone of voice and the anxiety expressed in the dialogue communicated the necessary information for me to help my student explore deeper issues in the client relationship and with the client's art expression. Now, many years later, I am studying the effects of virtual art therapy supervision and the differences between face-to-face, distant learning, and live-online supervision.

This chapter will cover the psychological effects of virtual art therapy interventions, such as through videoconferencing, which increased with the arrival of the COVID pandemic. I will examine the complex ideas of virtual art psychotherapy and its virtual healing qualities since "[i]n analytical psychotherapy ... the main pivot of treatment is transference. It is through the transference that affect, initially experienced in the past, is brought to 'live' into the present" (Schaverien, 1992, p. 1).

Just as Schaverien describes the transference of past experiences as being made "live," I will describe how virtual art therapy is "live-online." Following

DOI: 10.4324/9781003149538-13

Schaverien's investigations as "an exploration of the effects of the picture within the therapeutic relationship" (1992a [Abstract])—where the client, therapist, and artwork are located at the vertices of a relationship triangle—we are looking at the virtual triangle's therapeutic relationship with an added dimension, the fourth element of the computer screen. My colleague Winkel and I have conceptualized this as the squaring of the Schaverien triangle. I also hope to demonstrate how "the spiritual autonomy of the individual" (Cassirer as cited in Schaverien, 1992, p. 9) is maintained in virtual experiences.

Virtual Art Therapy Clinic

The COVID pandemic added a new challenge to art therapy due to the closures and lockdowns of many art therapy training schools and agencies where students planned to complete their practicum. The Virtual Art Therapy Clinic (VATC) of CiiAT was created in 2020 with two aims in mind:

- To provide accessible art therapy support to art therapy clients and to those members of the community at home and abroad, mentally affected by this world crisis
- To provide a virtual practicum setting for CiiAT students

With the introduction of https://arttherapy.network, the landing page of the VATC, CiiAT was faced with more questions than answers. The main questions for me and Winkel, the other lead clinic supervisor, revolved around therapeutic relationships and transference:

- Would it be possible to develop therapeutic relationships through videoconferencing?
- Would the therapist be aware of feelings of transference projected to the therapist and/or into the artwork?

I was amazed by the practicum students' presentations at supervision and their case studies. I will be using the students' work to illustrate this therapeutic phenomenon through case studies, vignettes, and illustrations generated during video-based art therapy sessions in the VATC. Included is client art and personal materials as well as art created on Zoom Whiteboard during sessions.

Transference in Art Therapy

For Schaverien, "the main pivot of treatment is transference" (1992, p. 11), which is often accompanied by an intense way of relating and offers "the opportunity for transformation" (p. 11). Transference is a Freudian concept explained by Charles Rycroft as the process by which a patient displaces on to his analyst feelings, ideas, etc., which derive from previous figures in his life; by which he relates to his analyst as though he were some former object in his life; by which he projects on to his analyst object-representations acquired by earlier introjections; by which he endows the analyst with the significance of another, usually prior, object.

(1985, p. 168)

The opposite effect is countertransference, which describes the analyst's transference on the client and can be a distorting element in treatment, considering emotional attitudes and responses towards particular client behaviors (Rycroft, 1985, p. 25). The therapist, however, "can use this latter kind of countertransference as clinical evidence; i.e., he can assume that his own emotional response is based on a correct interpretation of the patient's true intentions or meaning" (p. 25).

When describing transference in terms of an art therapy process, we are looking at

1   The process by which the client displaces onto the art therapist feelings, ideas, etc.
2   The process by which the client displaces onto the art product feelings, ideas, etc.
3   The therapeutic relationship that forms the triangle

In virtual art therapy, all of this is taking place on the computer screen, which adds a further element and conceptually squares the triangle. The same applies to delivering supervision online.

Virtual Supervision

Supervision has always been a vital part of art therapy training as it assists students to become effective art therapists and mental health professionals. Through comments and questions, the supervisor models for the trainee how to look at clinical material, how to avoid premature conclusions, and how to refrain from negative judgments about the client or the intervention used. Fenichel's (1997) supervision manual highlights the importance of reflective practice already "in preservice training, nurtured by mutually respectful relationships with instructors, fieldworks supervisors, and mentors" (p. 35), which not only supports therapy practice but also individualizes training experiences.

Supervision is how we teach art therapists to identify the concepts in their work with clients. In her book *A Traveler's Guide to Art Therapy Supervision* (2011), Monica Carpendale describes this process as

a pilgrimage of sorts—a wandering, a muddling along and circling to find a way into the center. The intention is to explore the process of supervision with a primary focus on the internal frame of reference with regards to the travelers' mind and the pattern of the unfolding journey of supervision.

(p.11)

Being an art therapist in training is a delicate and emotional space between one's own life experiences and that of the client. The art therapy trainee who works with a virtual platform has the added stress of delivering art therapy to clients in a new form, for which there are no books to read and no professional examples to follow. Thus, the art therapy trainee may doubt their value in delivering art therapy this way and must be fully supported through their practical training.

The supervisors are also going through an intensive learning experience, as virtual art therapy and virtual supervision are new to them as well. The therapist no longer controls the office in which they welcome the client, making sure it is safe, comfortable, and age appropriate. Similarly, the therapist no longer controls the art material that the client uses to express their pain and stress through art-making, which means they can no longer surprise the client with a new material to use, or introduce tactile materials to a 'resistant' client. Furthermore, if the client does not have an extra camera, the therapist often cannot follow the clients' movements on the page, the clients' body language, or the amount of softness or pressure that the client uses to create the image. Yet despite these restrictions, student art therapists have managed to reach and help many clients through the rectangular screen of the computer, mobile phone, or tablet. As the supervisor of many CiiAT students, I was delighted to see the art that was produced and the many creative ways the art therapist used to introduce therapeutic interventions.

The client now has control of the therapeutic space, oversees making it safe and confidential, and controls the media used in art expression, albeit with COVID-19 lockdown impediments to obtaining art supplies. When the art therapist wishes to introduce an intervention, they must ask the client to provide the necessary material.

Further points to consider for virtual sessions:

- How does the therapist manage someone else coming into the client's room, interrupting the session?
- How do we manage a client stating they have no art making materials?
- What do you do when the cat cozies up or the dog wants attention, or even more importantly, if a baby shows up in the space?
- What happens to the artwork—is it kept in a safe place? Is it respected?
- Will the client take photos and send them to their therapist?
- Can the therapist take screenshots without the client's permission?
- What has happened to our ethics, which we must follow religiously?
- What new codes of ethics are being created?

Thus, the art therapist must be prepared for unexpected circumstances that had never been anticipated during traditional training. As a supervisor, I am expecting that they use their creativity at those moments.

Over the past 30 years as an art therapy supervisor, I encouraged students to take copious notes and photos of the artwork and to keep this material for publication with the client's consent. This chapter will explore case studies of student art therapists working with children, adolescents, and adults. Some of the art was created with traditional art materials. Other pieces were created with non-traditional, household materials, such as spices or vegetables, while other clients incorporated personal items.

Marilyn Hahn—Working with a Talisman

Working virtually is a new situation for most established art therapists. The student art therapist, however, has the additional challenge that training resources, such as videos, focus on in-person sessions with clients, which means she does not have much guidance to figure out how virtual art therapy works. Nonetheless, CiiAT student art therapist Marilyn Hahn, after expressing her own frustrations at working virtually, was able to establish significant therapeutic relationships with her clients. Hahn has many years of experience working as a teacher with rebelling adolescents. She drew on her previous experience as an instructor with difficult students by using personal objects in therapy when her clients did not have art materials or refused to make art. In supervision, Hahn was able to understand the concepts of transference to the personal possession as an art expression.

Although unaware of the Schaverien concept of the Talisman, while working with a senior client who was objecting to using art materials, Hahn pointed to a large Ferris wheel photograph on the wall behind the client. In the discussion about the wheel, the client revealed significant information from her past. The Ferris wheel photograph became the Talisman, an object with powerful attachment (Schaverien, 1992), representing a significant memory in her client's life. The client was able to express feelings of the chaos in her life, of the freedom to fly, and a secure feeling of connectedness to her centre.

As a supervisor, I was able to understand the closeness of the therapeutic relationship. It was as if they had connected with each other as in an in-person session. Following this experience, Hahn encouraged her clients to open cupboards to look for art that they created a long time ago. Hahn felt that objects held an emotional story that was more powerful and easily elicited than by using traditional art materials. She found that epiphanies seemed more commonly experienced with possessions. Hahn further states that a possession is anything—material or immaterial—owned, lost, given away, stolen, damaged but meaningful enough to tell a story about the values of Self extended into the world so that others can see, touch, hear, and validate the Self.

This new type of virtual intervention, with the client sitting at home during a session, gave her a path into the psyche of her client, like an image of an object in their art. Hahn's work brings to mind the Schaverien concept of "The Talisman: the empowered picture" (1992, p. 137). The Talisman in Hahn's work becomes not only the empowered picture, but also the empowered personal possession.

Case Vignette 1—Marilyn Hahn

Client Mary depicted her feelings about a necklace in art making, which she identified as a stolen personal possession, by using gray-toned embossing powders, glue, and a heat gun on stiff paper. She experienced surprise at the face that emerged, immediately identifying it as both her naive adolescent self, forgiving the offenders, and her angry, resentful adult self (see Figure 10.1), admonishing both the child self and the offending clerics. After carefully reproducing the original necklace, somatically and intuitively choosing materials that elicited the same feelings as the original one (cold metal and dulled pearl), and then adding it to the art piece, Mary aggressively added swirls, lines, and smudges to the piece (see Figure 10.2), depicting the ever present, painful tension in her body and mind as clouds of unrelenting toxic thoughts, words, self-shaming, and regret.

After the session, she took a few days of emotional engagement with the art piece on her own, which included journalling and meditating, before she responded to the question asked in the session, "What's missing in this art piece?" She admitted to struggling with the question until she removed the necklace, immediately sensing then that, to her, the necklace represented being choked: a tightness in her body as a blockage that prevented her from releasing negativity. In addition, she decided that love and peace were missing. She then added three hearts and a dove in the scribble-drawn swirls (see Figure 10.3). With the conscious removal of the necklace and the deliberate addition of colour and symbols to the otherwise dark piece, Mary indicated that an

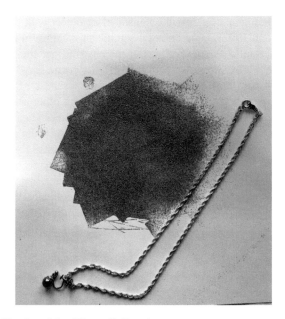

Figure 10.1 The Anguish of Turmoil: Part 1

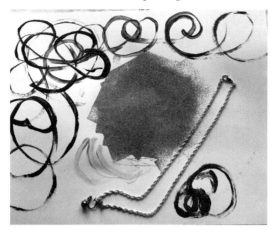

Figure 10.2 The Anguish of Turmoil: Part 2

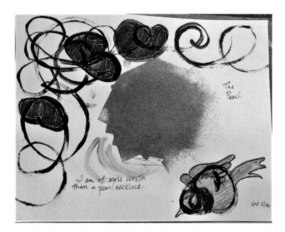

Figure 10.3 The Addition of Love and Peace

expansive feeling of relief and lightness engulfed her. The story of the taken necklace no longer held the grip it once had.

In her case analysis, Hahn suggested that Mary created a new reality for herself by fully engaging in art-making. Mary indicated a surprise at the ease with which she interacted with her personal possession despite past triggers of anger and shame when thinking of the original necklace or holding the reproduction.

Case Vignette 1—Discussion

During my supervision with Hahn, we were able to identify the transference Mary held to this piece of jewelry that she felt had been stolen. The fact that the client had the impression that it was choking her was a significant negative transference, which I described using Schaverien's concept as a scapegoat transference. In this type of transference, the artwork becomes the embodied scapegoat. With her art therapy skills, Hahn was able to get the client to add peace and love to the drawing, which helped dissolve the negative emotions enmeshed in this piece of jewelry.

Making these connections to personal possessions is a process not easily done in face-to-face therapy. Granted, a client could go home to find an object and bring it back to the office. This, however, lacks the experience of the client finding the possession during the session and keeping it with them in their own space.

The space, the place where the therapy happens, is always sacred. When that space is in the home of the client, it remains sacred. It is the process and the skills of the art therapist that will allow this space to remain a peaceful and trusting space to occupy. Interacting with the pseudo, but still powerful, necklace helped craft a story of love, peace, and self-determination, as well as freedom from recurring negative thoughts about choking, and an increased sense of wellbeing and healing.

When we discuss transference and countertransference in art therapy, we talk about the emotional process that occurs from the client to the therapist and to the artwork. These transferences have the effect of drawing the therapist—and at times the supervisor—into the image. These processes apply differently when working with children, as the following section shows.

Supervision for Art Therapy Students Working Virtually with Children

In the above section, I have been focusing on discovering the transference and countertransference in the sessions. We will also be alert for these concepts when working with children, but these will mostly be apparent through the child's interaction with the therapist. Regularly, the artwork of children will not depict imagery that contains underlying emotional issues. To reach these levels, the art therapist may use role playing, third person interpretation, interactive play, or toys.

Working virtually with children requires the help of the parent in order to prepare the space, supply the materials, and set up the meeting through Zoom. The parent is, therefore, much more involved in virtual art therapy than they would be if the child were coming to the therapist in-person. It is exceedingly difficult to keep the art products confidential, as the parent may be the one responsible to keep it in a safe place at home. This is the great advantage of the Zoom Whiteboard, where art expressions are digital and have a greater possibility of remaining private.

The following section presents insights submitted to this chapter by Aditi Kaul. Kaul is a psychologist and UNESCO and CID certified creative arts therapist utilizing Dance Movement Therapy. This vignette highlights the value of artwork created on the Zoom Whiteboard.

Aditi Kaul—Virtual Art Therapy Sessions

Exploring the Zoom Whiteboard throughout 2020, Kaul found that not only was this digital, art-making tool effective with teenagers, but she was also able to work with children older than five years, as well as adults. Some of the younger children she worked with felt extremely trapped in the initial months of the pandemic lockdown and shared their fears around the illness, their own safety, and boredom. The Whiteboard became a tool to escape lockdown confinement, to virtually play in the park, run, jump, be angry, and express frustration, and to build narratives by saving, erasing, and logging what they created.

Figure 10.4 was made by a six-year-old boy who began bed-wetting and having panic attacks in the middle of the night. This is an excerpt from the third session in which he created his favourite park and asked Kaul to help draw certain figures that he would then edit or correct. He would scribble out a swing and say, "Don't touch," plan a picnic where they would add food, and then remove it once they had eaten.

Kaul found that the art process lent itself to play. It allowed them to work on one collective image, enabling a strong sense of inhabiting the same room. The parents were happy with the use of the Whiteboard, as they had to make no monetary investment in collecting art media and yet the results were powerful. Kaul was able to integrate music in the background where needed and also saw her young clients jump in excitement when they communicated exactly how they felt, or when they crossed paths in an on-screen scribble game but their lines appeared with a one-second delay as a surprise. The scribble technique, a quick and playful joint drawing activity to help the client relieve stress and begin art therapy, typically used on paper, now came to life on the Whiteboard. It presented them with the opportunity to play discover, retain the artwork, but then also redraw and explore boundaries after reflecting on what had emerged. This technique worked with children, adolescents, and adults alike.

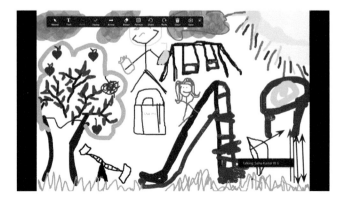

Figure 10.4 Favourite Park

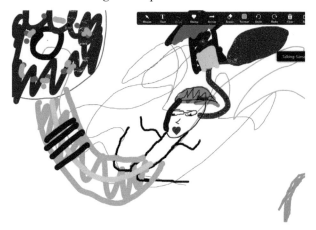

Figure 10.5 Scribble Drawing: Party Gone Mad (13-Year-Old Client)

While watching people's narratives unfold, re-enacting and altering trauma events, Kaul learnt that the Whiteboard could be a transformational platform encompassing the core concepts of play (used in trauma work with children) and visual art. When used with adults, the Whiteboard allowed for the intersection of play and art without triggering their defenses about doing something "silly" or playing with "toys."

Case Vignette 2—Aditi Kaul

Client Light first stepped into Kaul's office in 2018 with her mother with a presenting problem of anxiety. She was a quiet, cautious, and observant 10-year old,

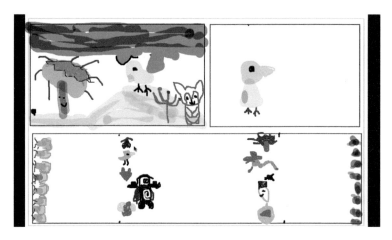

Figure 10.6 Narratives in Play

and slowly, through art, began to open up. She was being bullied, had thoughts of self-harm, and difficulties with her mood. After a year of art therapy, she had better interpersonal relationships, support systems, and an improved understanding of herself.

When COVID-19 hit in 2020, schools closed and her parents reached out to restart therapy online. In the first session, Kaul and Light co-created art physically across the screen, but Light seemed disconnected, irritable, and more focused on defense-filled verbalization than art making. In session 2, Kaul decided to try the Zoom Whiteboard with Light, asking her to play and begin creating. Light immediately embraced the tool and created an image that she named "floating noodles."

For the first couple of sessions, they had absolute silence as Light created a new world and narrative for herself. Characters emerged, and for the first time in Kaul's career, she saw the art process grow with a client on a screen. Kaul witnessed the client's frustration and anger, her laughter as a stroke emerged that made her happy, and what she chose to erase and redo.

The conversation was carried out purely through colours and her characters, which started with the noodle face, grew into Jan, Januy, Pete Wenstand, and finally the central characters of Dill and the man from the band "Panic at The Disco." The narrative centred around Dill, who was strong, steadfast, and someone she called a "star" who would stand up for what he believed in.

Light simultaneously began sharing about a boy with whom she would have "fun fights and banter" and narrated a very enmeshed relationship built solely on music with three new friends. As the sessions progressed, Kaul supported her in building the narrative as they continued with her characters on the Whiteboard. She introduced a blood splatter that transformed to ketchup and other condiments for support as Brendon (the man from "Panic at the Disco") planned his revenge. As Dill's friend stabbed him in the back as part of what she described as a violent kill, her anger found a voice.

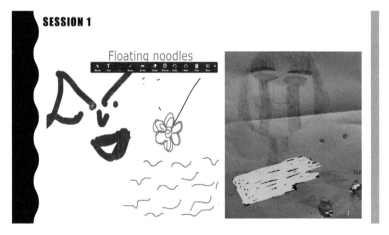

Figure 10.7 Session 1: Artwork with Floating Noodles Image

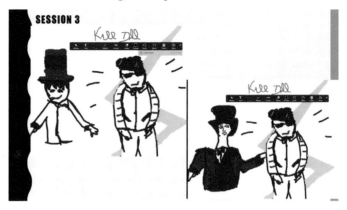

Figure 10.8 Session 3: Artwork with Dill Character

With increasing violence and abstraction, Light was pushing Kaul's boundaries. Kaul could see the anger in the strokes, feel her own heart race, and countertransferential feelings build. Kaul felt an urge to know and understand what had happened to Light and who had hurt her.

Two weeks later, as the artwork and narrative progressed to Dill transformed into a pile of poop, Light shared that her three new friends were cyberbullying her. Kaul saw the light begin to leave Light as she struggled week after week with the same image, creating different versions, with arrows, colours, and additions. Finally, she said to Kaul, "I think I'm done with Dill because poop goes back into the earth. This helps plants grow!" This moment, in which she shared how the poop would be able to grow back, was a sign of her strength. This paralleled her narrative of finally beginning to cut off ties with the three friends who had persistently bullied her, even though she had tried to be assertive and communicate what she needed. It showed the value of using the Whiteboard in her healing process, permitting a narrative she could rework over and over, which would have taken many hours to do on paper. "Can you feel the glass smashing?" she said when she hit the *redo* and *undo* buttons, creating motion in her art.

The middle narrative that surfaced was about pee, toilet paper, and revenge. She created art in which, yet again, Kaul could feel the client trying to push her away, to get a reaction, which mirrored recent arguments and fights Light had with her mother. The transference grew as Light quickly deleted the art before Kaul had a chance to save it and then laughed and brought it back up. The process allowed the client to enact transferential feelings with power and autonomy. At some points, Kaul felt the urge to yell, or simply log off when Light would randomly turn off her camera or mute herself.

Through an art review, Light was able to verbally connect and share for the first time what she thought the characters stood for. She wanted to stab her

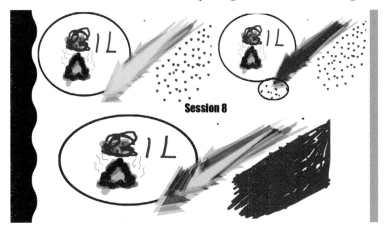

Figure 10.9 Session 8: Artwork with Poop Images

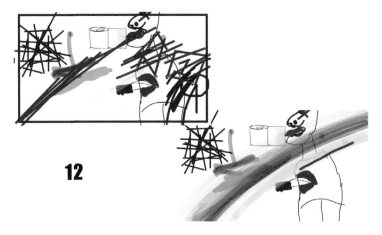

Figure 10.10 Session 11: Middle Narrative Artwork

friends in the art, and did so vicariously through the narrative. She asked Kaul if they could continue using the Whiteboard even when they would meet in person in the future. When Kaul asked her why, Light said that it gave her a voice and more freedom than she had ever felt on paper.

The final image was a large cut with stitches on it. Even though it was simplistic, she spent time making it exactly how she wanted. When she finished the last stitch, both therapist and client exhaled simultaneously, and Kaul felt an exaggerated sense of attunement with Light and the artwork. They had seen a marked shift in her confidence, assertiveness, sense of autonomy, range of emotional expression, and sense of self.

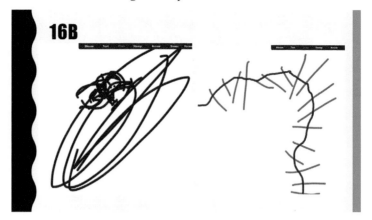

Figure 10.11 Session 16: Artwork with Stitches Image

Case Vignette 2—Discussion

The Whiteboard allowed the client to do and undo marks, allowing her to express her unconscious and conscious feelings. The art therapist released the power of the image by acknowledging and supporting it, which allowed the art play to express transference as well as elicit countertransference in Kaul. By recognizing her own countertransference, Kaul was able to begin to understand the underlying emotions expressed in the artwork and client. Therefore, in this case study, we see how virtual art therapy and the use of the Whiteboard allowed a 10-year-old preadolescent to trust the therapist, allowing her to feel free to express repressed negative and positive emotions.

Kaul adds:

> As a practicing therapist for over nine years now, to use a full-fledged virtual medium, something that we never learnt about in our books, is an example of the revolutionary power of creativity and how, when we struggle with less, we are often able to access more—more ideas, more insights, and newer resources to tap into. In a country like India, where we still have a significant shortage of mental health professionals, the Whiteboard gave me the ability to work with clients across the country and the world. Some managed to access the tool from remote areas on their phones to experience art therapy. I found that we utilize art, language, movement, and shape our interventions with clients by starting with the medium that seems like the most comfortable extension of the self. For so many today, using technology has become part of their comfort language.

Conclusion

The interaction with clients through virtual means provides the therapists with new opportunities, such as meeting clients in their own space or allowing a digital method, like the Zoom Whiteboard, for clients to create art without having to buy art materials. Transference and countertransference experienced in virtual sessions with adults and children show that this mobilization of affect is also present in the virtual therapeutic relationship. For instance, Zoom Whiteboard enables the therapist to watch clients create digital art and observe client's projections and transference onto characters in the artwork. However, there are also challenges, such as clients having the power to end sessions by simply cutting the connection. Virtual art therapy redefines the relationship and interaction between client and therapist, and art therapy organizations, like the Canadian Art Therapy Association, are slowly setting up new rules around ethical questions when providing therapy online. The use of the Schaverien Talisman and Scapegoat concepts can be applied in a more intimate way by meeting clients virtually at their own home. Thus, with the added virtual element to therapy, we are squaring the Schaverien triangle.

References

Carpendale, M. (2011). *A traveler's guide to art therapy supervision.* Trafford Publishers: Canada.

Fenichel, E. E. (1997). *Learning through supervision and mentorship to support the development of infants, toddlers and their families: A source book. National Center for Infants, Toddlers and Families.* Zero to Three/National Center for Clinical Infant Programs: Washington, DC.

Rycroft, C. (1985). *A critical dictionary of psychoanalysis.* Penguin Books: London and New York.

Schaverien, J. (1992). *The revealing image: Analytical art psychotherapy in theory and practice.* Routledge: London and New York.

Schaverien, J. (1992a). *The revealing image: Analytical art psychotherapy in theory and practice.* Routledge: London and New York. Abstract retrieved from https://psycnet.apa.org/record/1993-97886-000.

11 Evolution of a Virtual Art Therapy Open Studio

Sheila Lorenzo de la Peña and Carolyn Brown Treadon

Introduction

The origins of an open studio model in art therapy can be traced back to the beginning of the profession (Finkel & Bat Or, 2020; Moon, 2016). This approach has the capacity to foster an individual's ability to be alone while in the presence of another, a concept developed by Winnicott (Finkel & Bat Or, 2020), which can lead to increased emotional maturity and enable individuals to better integrate into social and community spaces. It gathers individuals into a collective space, often those living outside of the mainstream, who have limited access to other mental health resources (Kapitan, 2008).

The fully online graduate art therapy program at Edinboro University, PA, developed an open studio space as a way to create in-person connections for faculty, staff, and students. When the global pandemic began in 2020, the open studio needed to move online as well, which created new challenges. This chapter explores the historical roots of the open studio in art therapy, modern uses, Edinboro University's approach to a campus-based open studio, and the shift to a virtual platform following the closure of the community studio space.

Historical Context for the Open Studio

In the early 1930s, Mary Huntoon was hired as an artist to provide instruction at Winter VA Hospital, which was part of the Menninger Clinic in Topeka, Kansas (Finkel & Bat Or, 2020; Moon, 2016). She established a studio space where patients could engage in artistic expression, which she believed had therapeutic value. Similarly, Edward Adamson, an artist in the United Kingdom, was hired as an arts master in 1946 for Netherene Psychiatric Hospital to establish an open studio (Finkel & Bat Or, 2020). Adamson later connected with Adrian Hill who had been working in a sanitorium for individuals recovering from tuberculosis. Hill, an artist, used art to work through his own recovery and continued to provide art groups at the hospital where he saw the benefits of art to increase wellness and aid in healing (Bush, n.d.). Allen (2008) postulated that healing in a group comes from navigating the inherent

DOI: 10.4324/9781003149538-14

struggle in art making alongside others experiencing similar challenges. Through the open studio, relationships develop between the participants and within each individual as everyone experiences a shared engagement in the "stuff of life" (Allen, 2008, p. 11).

Primary Features of an Open Studio

Moon (2016) discussed that the open studio has an informal, dynamic atmosphere where the focus is on health over pathology. The role of the art therapist is seen as less hierarchical and more flexible—sometimes maintaining safety and assisting when needed, and at other times creating alongside participants. They carry the belief that all individuals have the innate ability to be creative (Ottemiller & Awais, 2016). Thus, an open structure creates an environment that is conducive to creative expression where the focus is on the process and the product, with neither more important than the other.

In an effort to understand if there were increased benefits for an art therapy open studio with participants who had prior art knowledge, Kaimal and Ray (2016) conducted a study to compare positive and negative affect and self-efficacy with individuals who had prior art-making experience and those who did not. Results indicated that there were no significant differences between participants. Participation in a single session of art making led to an overall increase in positive affect, a decrease in negative affect, and increased feelings of self-efficacy. In a follow-up, Kaimal et al. (2017) compared changes in affect, self-efficacy, and creative agency between individuals who participated in an art therapy open studio and those who were only provided a coloring page. Both groups experienced an increase in positive affect and a decrease in negative affect and stress, but the participants in the open studio reported a significant increase in positive affect—as well as self-efficacy—and creative agency. These results (Kaimal & Ray, 2016; Kaimal et al., 2017) indicate the potential of the art therapy open studio to increase overall health and wellness across the lifespan.

Open Studio in Art Therapy Education

Crane and Byrne (2020) explored the use of the open studio in art therapy education as a third space. Timm-Bottos and Reilly (2015) describe the third space as "complex environments that have transformative potential" (p. 103). In this space, education can be put into practice in a safe and guided way. It is a place where the teaching alliance can be extended through mentorship, challenging students, and the creation of an in-between space (Crane & Byrne 2020; Timm-Bottos & Reilly, 2015). This in-between state incorporates who students are and who they will become, a place to work through personal struggles and form professional identities. Working with clients places students in a situation to better understand themselves and how their lived experience impacts interactions while they receive supervision and mentorship to navigate the formation of new identities that reconcile with their past.

Development of a Virtual Open Studio

Initially, the graduate art therapy program at Edinboro University, PA, created an in-person open studio to provide a space for students, staff, faculty, and community members to benefit from art therapy for personal wellness. Participation was voluntary and on a weekly drop-in basis. A faculty member and graduate assistant staffed the space. As a fully online art therapy program, the faculty and students sought to create in-person opportunities for community building—the open studio was such a place.

The transition to the digital space was evolving before the pandemic of 2020 forced global communities to flood every corner of the digital landscape. We had discussed moving the studio online as a viable means of creating community for our 100% online Master's program. Our goal was to create a virtual space where students could come together and create, without judgment or pressure of an assignment, and build community. The pandemic merely hastened the implementation timeline not only for us, but many others as well.

The digital framework served as an access point; it does not preclude participants from the coveted sensory experiences of art making. We saw the transition to a virtual studio as a needed modification of service delivery. A recent graduate shared that it was not until the virtual studio that they felt connected to their peers and the program. They expressed sadness that it was not available until the pandemic and encouraged us to keep it running even after things returned to 'normal.'

Community Building in the Virtual Studio

Miller (2018) wrote that "the collective spirit seeks joining and attachment to community" (p.75). She enumerated how digital communities can be useful for art therapy students, post-graduates, established art therapists, as well as seasoned and retired professionals. While one of the initial reasons for providing the virtual studio was to build community for the art therapy students as a place to connect with peers and continue to develop their artist identities, our concept of community has expanded. Within a few months of hosting the virtual studios, we saw recent graduates attending as a way to stay connected to creative practices as well as to a community of support. Art-therapy-program graduates would often share some of their successes, struggles, and tips with other attendees.

After the virtual studio was shared on an American Art Therapy Association (AATA) blog, we began to see experienced and retired art therapists in attendance, often seeking a place in which to reconnect with their creative practice and like-minded individuals. Art therapists were by no means the only attendees of the virtual studio. In the spirit of the traditional studio, our virtual studio was open to all ages and professional affiliations. The number of participants, while not limited, was ideally 6–12 participants per studio.

As the pandemic continued, the virtual studio was shared with various groups of potential users (i.e. AATA blog, Facebook, Instagram, Eventbrite, course classrooms, and by personal email). The number of studio sessions offered varied each semester depending on the number of practicum and internship students allocated to the project. Some semesters we had as few as three studios per week and as high as six per week. All studios followed the same basic guidelines and lasted about two hours.

Considerations for a Virtual Studio

Similar to face-to-face studios, "individuals connect to digital communities at their own discretion and choosing" (Miller, 2018, p. 77). As such, the virtual studio is an ever-changing digital space that is constantly adapting to the needs of its users and facilitators. Due to its digital nature, these changes are easier to make and are more set-in-place than in a traditional studio. For instance, facilitators could run the studio from their home versus having to travel during inclement weather. Furthermore, they could continue holding the virtual studio when there are emergency regulations in place that limit face-to-face events. After a full year of hosting virtual studios, Table 11.1 on the following page highlights some items to consider.

The facilitator or lead is at the centre of the studio space. They hold the space by providing structure (a clear beginning, middle, end), setting the tone (provide a prompt and leads by example of how and what to share), providing primary support (validating participant experiences and promoting creative engagement), troubleshooting (technology and media), and redirecting participants as needed (if someone shares potentially triggering content). In essence, the facilitator leads by example. They make art synchronously and speak about it with the group in a way that models boundaries and effective use of creative expression in the service of emotional processing. Leads need to have the experience to understand and maintain healthy boundaries and the authority to make the call and remove a participant from the space if they must. They need to understand the digital interface and have a grasp on basic technical troubleshooting, and they also need to know whom to contact for last minute support.

In general, the virtual studios are scheduled for a two-hour block of time. Participants can come in any time after the studio is opened by the facilitator (not before). In cases where safety is of concern, a pre-identified "doors-close" time could be implemented. When the lead closes the meeting, no new participants can join. At times, the studio may close early especially if participation is low, and everyone finishes early.

All our studios follow the same format. They have a set day of the week and a set time frame. Facilitators welcome the attendees as they arrive and provide brief instructions, such as "We'll get started in ten minutes, go ahead and gather your supplies." Once the studio begins in earnest (which could be five minutes or ten minutes after the start time) the facilitator introduces the space, what it is for (creating art for wellness and uplifting each other), and

Table 11.1 Considerations for the Studio

	Considerations	Example
Purpose	1. What is the purpose of hosting the studio? 2. Who is the studio for?	1. Overall purpose is to host a space for community building through creative engagement—for wellness 2. Studio is open to everyone
Roles	1. Who will be the studio lead(s)? 2. Will there be a supervisor or other line of command/report? 3. What is the expectation for the participants?	1. Studio will be led by graduate art therapy students in practicum courses. Back-up leads will be filled by current graduate assistants in the art therapy program 2. Studio will be supervised by a full-time art therapy faculty 3. Participants are not expected to have an art background nor to have supplies
Safety	1. How will safety of participants and studio lead be implemented and maintained? 2. What is the follow-up to failed safety measures or transgressions?	1. Studio leads will be trained in basic platform safety. On Zoom that means how to be Host, lock a meeting, silence, remove participants, etc. 2. When a malicious event occurs, leads are to take control of the space, then notify supervisor. Follow-up with those present who witnessed the malicious event, but were not involved for processing. Post event attempt is made at locating information on removed participants and local authorities informed. Work with authorities as needed. Process with all studio leads and improve safety measures.
Guidelines	1. What structure will the studio have? Duration? Pace? Rules? Will each studio mirror the other or not?	1. All studios will follow a similar structure as follows (duration 2hrs): Intro (with music if possible), introduction of theme, art making time (with music), discussion, close. Simple guidelines are provided at each studio on expectations such as: Be willing to try new ideas/concepts, practice listening, right to pass (not share).

what it is not for (not for therapy or discussion of graphic or triggering content). Participants are then encouraged to introduce themselves and, if they wish, share what brought them to the studio. As introductions wind down to a close, the facilitator introduces a theme or guiding topic for the session. Usually, themes are open-ended so participants can interpret it for themselves and use whatever means they have available for creative processing. Recently a studio theme related to illustrating-identifying "your passion," further explained as those things that are a part of you that fuel you even if they are sometimes difficult or challenging to manage. Some drew hearts and added words, most explored the theme with abstract representations, and at least one created a soft sculpture using felt pieces she found in her room.

Studio themes serve to organize the facilitator and the space. The themes have a strong mental wellness and mental health relationship and are always optional. After the theme is discussed and tailored to the needs of the group, which is done on the spot, the facilitator designates the time for active art making, usually no less than 45 minutes and sometimes as long as an hour-and-a-half. They explain that music will be playing in the background and, in case someone needs to mute the sound, they give a stop time that allows for a closing discussion (15–30 minutes from the end time).

After the art making time has passed, the facilitator transitions the group into the closing discussion. In a similar fashion to the studio opening, a brief statement is given about the purpose of the closing discussion and some parameters or guidelines are refreshed. Participants are reminded that speaking about their piece or showing it to the group is optional. The facilitator will then either open the floor for sharing or be the first to share to set an example for how and how much to share. Participants are invited to contribute to the discussion by means of either sharing the work they made or providing commentary—neither is expected, but both are welcome.

Facilitators are coached and encouraged to use music as placeholders for 'in-between' times, such as when participants wait to begin or when art making is taking place. This is especially useful during the 45–90 minutes of art making when eye contact breaks with the group and everyone creates in their spaces. Playing music helps the group feel as if they are still connected and can help cue a return to the group space once the music is stopped. It is important to listen to the potential music selections prior to their introduction to the studio and consider the impact that certain music choices can have on the creative process. Facilitators can also inform participants about using their own music and muting the studio's audio selection. We assume participants have at least a rudimentary understanding of the internet and their device. On the part of the facilitator, they must be comfortable with the technology and devices being used.

An area for consideration when it comes to safety is being transparent that the studio is not group therapy. This involves an understanding that emotions may flare, as the creative process may tap into unforeseen corners of our psyche. The lead needs to be able to redirect or help the participant become grounded once again. Since the virtual studios we hold are accessible from around the world, it is a challenge to provide local access to assistance if it were to be needed. What we have done so far is compile a list of national and international helplines that is accessible to the studio facilitators if they were to need it. The supervising faculty and peers (i.e. other studio leads) are also accessible through a shared chat, such as Microsoft Teams or a similar application, for support and troubleshooting.

The following section provides an example of how the virtual studio was utilized and adapted for the benefit of a group seeking a creative outlet for socialization and creative expression. In the example, the virtual studio continued to foster the main concept of art for wellness, but in order to prioritize the participants' safety, the group was held in a closed group format outside of regular studio sessions.

Virtual Creative Journaling Group for Adolescents

Seven girls, aged 12–15, participated in a 6-week closed group along with 2 facilitators. The participants were struggling due to isolation and missed peer interactions. Each member of the group was provided a starter kit that included a journal, markers, coloured pencils, glue, watercolour paint, pencils, and an eraser. They were encouraged to also bring any other materials they had at home to the virtual studio.

The group met for 90 minutes once a week. Each week, participants engaged in a check-in, identifying one thing they had done during the past week that was fun or exciting. The check-ins allowed those who did not know each other to connect. After the first week, participants were encouraged to work in their journals in-between sessions. Following the first session, where participants decorated their journals, they were asked to bring collage materials to the next group to create an image to represent themselves. When asked to explain their image, one participant explained, "This journaling page uses watercolor and magazine cutouts to express my hobbies and passions in a creative way" (see Figure 11.1 and 11.2).

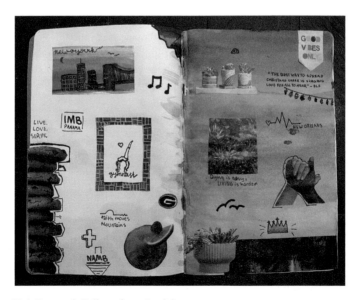

Figure 11.1 Personal Collage from Participant

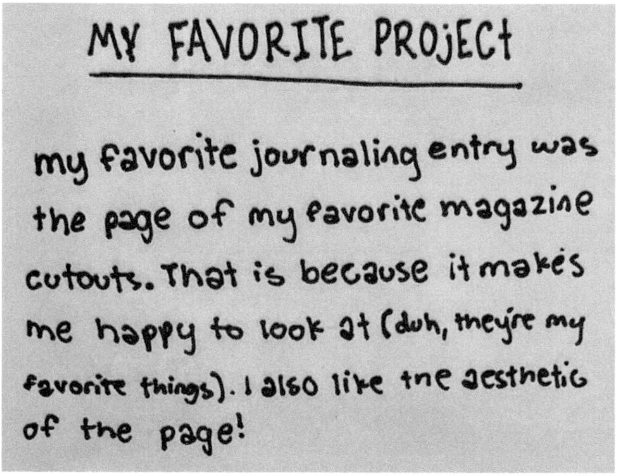

MY FAVORITE PROJECT

my favorite journaling entry was
the page of my favorite magazine
cutouts. That is because it makes
me happy to look at (duh, they're my
favorite things). I also like the aesthetic
of the page!

Figure 11.2 Participant Explanation of Her Favourite Project

Future prompts included finding a piece of art they were drawn to in a virtual museum or a book to share with the group, one thing you wish people knew about you, a quote or image you find inspirational, coping skills you use, and how you think others see you and how you want to be seen.

Figure 11.3 was one participant's response to an inspirational message. She stated that

> this is my favourite journal entry. I chose this one because I love the colour purple! Also, each of these sayings that are listed represents me and who I am. Another reason why I think this page is unique [is that] each strip of purple is different with the textures and colours.

Another reported that "identifying what makes me unique was my favourite entry. We made a list as a group and then picked out the words that meant the most to us" (Figure 11.4).

Participants reported that they enjoyed the group because it allowed them a social outlet and the opportunity to meet new people. One participant shared that "I really enjoyed this program because it was a fun way to socialize and make new friends while in quarantine." The participants expressed sadness when the group ended, stating it was nice to have something to look forward to each week. One participant shared she had plans for continuing to use her journal as self-care and had created a list of ideas for future entries (see Figure 11.5).

Conclusion

From the early beginning of art therapy, the open studio has served as an outlet for creative expression (Finkel & Bat Or, 2020). A return to this approach represents a

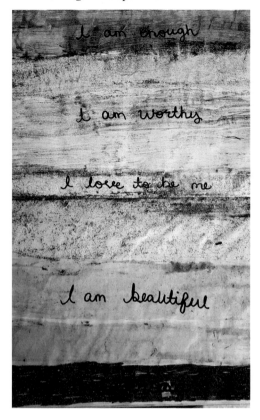

Figure 11.3 Participant's Response to an Inspirational Message

homecoming. Operating from a strengths-based perspective and focusing on wellness represents a shift away from pathologizing clients. It takes the focus away from providing services to individuals to one of building community, where individuals support each other (Ottemiller & Awais, 2016). The creative process becomes the focus of the open studio. In its innate flexibility, the open studio increases accessibility to diverse populations in a multitude of settings (Finkel & Bat Or, 2020, p. 8, p. 10). Expanding the definition of what art therapy can be creates an opportunity for a more inclusive and compassionate profession that has the potential to decrease stigma associated with mental health care, keeping social engagement at a primary focus (Allen, 2008; Moon, 2016, Ottemiller & Awais, 2016).

As a profession, we must think outside the box of what art therapy must look like to meet the needs of our communities. The virtual studio is one attempt to broaden the scope of practice to reach individuals who may not otherwise have access to art therapy. What started out as a programmatic opportunity for students has quickly grown to a service utilized by individuals around the globe to connect, create, and belong.

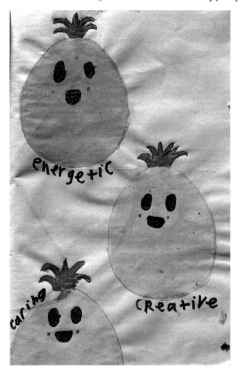

Figure 11.4 My Unique Qualities

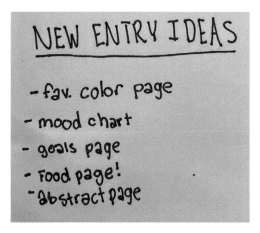

Figure 11.5 Journal for Self-Care: Future Plans

References

Allen, P. B. (2008). Commentary on community-based art studios: Underlying principles. *Art Therapy: Journal of the American Art Therapy Association, 25*, 11–12. doi: doi:10.1080/07421656.2008.10129350.

Bush, M. (n.d.). Adrien Hill: UK founder of art therapy. London Art Therapy Center. https://arttherapycentre.com/blog/adrian-hill-uk-founder-art-therapy-morgan-bush-intern/.

Crane, T., & Byrne, L. (2020). Risk, rupture, and change: Exploring the liminal space of the Open Studio in art therapy education. *The Arts in Psychotherapy, 69*. https://doi.org/10.1016/j.aip.2020.101666.

Finkel, D., & Bat Or, M. (2020) The open studio approach to Art Therapy: A systematic scoping Review. *Frontiers in Psychology, 11*. doi:10.3389/fpsyg.2020.568042.

Kaimal, G., & Ray, K. (2016). Free art-making in an art therapy open studio: Changes in affect and self-efficacy. *Arts & Health: International Journal for Research, Policy & Practice, 9*(2), 154–166. doi:10.1080/17533015.2016.1217248.

Kaimal, G., Mensinger, J. L., Drass, J. M., & Dieterich-Hartwell, R. M. (2017). Art therapist-facilitated open studio versus coloring: Differences in outcomes of affect, stress, creative agency, and self-efficacy. *Canadian Art Therapy Association Journal, 30*(2), 56–68. https://doi.org/10.1080/08322473.2017.1375827.

Kapitan, L. (2008). "Not art therapy": Revisiting the therapeutic studio in the narrative of the profession. *Art Therapy: Journal of the American Art Therapy Association, 25*(1), 2–3.

Miller, G. (2018). *The art therapist's guide to social media: Connection, community, and creativity*. Routledge.

Moon, C. (2016). Open studio approach to art therapy. In Gussak, D., Rosal, M. (eds.) *The Wiley Handbook of Art Therapy*. Wiley and Sons.

Ottemiller, D. D., & Awais, Y. J. (2016). A Model for Art Therapists in Community-Based Practice. *Art Therapy, 33*(3), 144–150.

Timm-Bottos, J., & Reilly, R. (2015). Learning in third spaces: Community art studio as storefront university classroom. *American Journal of Community Psychology, 55*(1–2), 102–114.

12 Cameras Off, Coffee On

Online Teaching and Learning in COVID-Times

Michele D. Rattigan

Introduction

As an instructor at Drexel University in Philadelphia, PA, U.S., I prepared to teach the course *Creativity, Symbolism, and Metaphor in Art Therapy and Counseling* that relied on art-based experientials. I had taught the course as an in-person experience since 2013, but had to adapt it to an online format with contact restrictions due to COVID-19. Some of the course objectives included that students would understand the connection of historical antecedents with contemporary practices and demonstrate specific properties and effects of art processes and materials informed by current research, such as the Expressive Therapies Continuum (Hinz, 2020; Kagin & Lusebrink, 1978). The challenge for me to teach a course online that was designed to be taught face-to-face and synchronous, was to be unafraid to deconstruct without compromising rigor and without causing harm and undo stress during the pandemic. I strived to support students' learning and hold the space without force; hence, all synchronous meetings for this class were optional. I was both surprised and grateful that this optional time had close to full attendance each week.

Our academic institution had initially planned to conduct a few weeks online, then a transition "back to normal" when possible. Once the 2020 spring quarter was underway, it became clear that any transition back to in-person learning would be delayed beyond any of our comfort levels. Knowing the learners and knowing the realities of their learning environments is imperative (Conrad & Donaldson, 2004), which leads to the instructor standing "ready to adjust activities as the needs of the community dictate" (Conrad & Donaldson, 2004, p. 19). Students do not learn in a vacuum, and the same holds true in an online format as this chapter will discuss.

Teaching in a Pandemic

My teaching philosophy focuses on the dynamic teacher–student relationship and presence as andragogy/pedagogy. I believe the teacher–student relationship in clinical education is a valuable tool to model and stimulate the basic foundations of healing that are taught in the human service professions. One

DOI: 10.4324/9781003149538-15

of these foundations is "therapeutic presence." Teaching therapeutic presence involves a combination of mindfulness of both teacher and student, students' self-reflective work, faculty modelling, and an intentional delivery of educational material from course conceptualization to imparting of information.

I found that constructivist learning theory aligned with my philosophy of teaching and adapted well when needing to teach online. Constructivist theory (Taylor & Hamdy, 2013) parallels my goal to assist students in navigating, organizing, and assimilating a vast amount of complex intra- and interpersonal material learning in classroom and clinical settings. It is not uncommon for some students to experience a complete reordering of their existence during in-vivo clinical activities in which learners shift from passive observers to active therapeutic facilitators (Dennick, 2012). This requires students to check themselves for biases and construct new understandings of themselves and the world (Dennick, 2012). Bruner (cited in Dennick, 2012) proposed the visual of a spiral to explain the constructivist element where students can 'circle back' to previously known material, build on it, and carry the spiral forward as they construct new learning. I've witnessed students not only monitor their own growth but compare themselves to their peers as much as they compare textbook theories to what they witness in the field.

One example to facilitate and encourage recognition of newly constructed knowledge in a tangible way is weekly image and text journals using response art (Fish, 2019), which can be facilitated online using a journal application. For instance, the BlackBoard learning management system has an application for journals that is confidential between the student and instructor. Students can write directly into the platform and attach documents, links, images, and short videos.

The elements I could pull from my teaching philosophy included being present and building connections while leaning into radical self-compassion (Brach, 2019; Brookfield, 1990). "Appearing confused, hesitant, or baffled seems a sign of weakness. And admitting that we feel tired, unmotivated, or bored seems a betrayal of the humanitarian zest we [teachers] are supposed to exhibit" (Brookfield, 1990, p. 3). Keeping this in mind, I "forgave" myself for not getting to all the nuggets of wisdom I hoped to impart and for not offering the same educational experiences that previous cohorts had.

The Art Coffeehouse

The art coffeehouse was a weekly synchronous offering of the course that occurred for one and half hours: half of the time that we would have typically spent together on the same day had we been allowed face-to-face instruction. While there was some pressure from the institution to "hold" synchronous meetings just like an in-person class, I resisted. I encouraged students to attend the synchronous meetings as much as possible, but the meetings were not mandatory, and students' grades would not be negatively impacted if they didn't attend. I was also clear that even if self-selecting to join, participation did not mandate their physical presence on camera nor were they expected to speak. Our time was what it needed to be. It was organic.

Students created their own structure in synchronous meetings. One week, a student shared a riddle and their peers requested they bring another one the following week. At other times, students asked questions about what they were reading asynchronously and how I may have experienced similar instances in my clinical practice. Some moments were spent troubleshooting technological mishaps with some of the digital asynchronous activities. Students asked each other about the art they were making for the ongoing course project and video tours were given of each other's working spaces and materials. Pets made frequent guest appearances. Some shared appreciation for the recorded slideshow lectures I built specifically for the course. One student disclosed that the recorded lectures were very helpful in navigating their learning and attention difficulties. Several students chimed in with agreement that they appreciated having control over the material: when to take it in, to be able to replay parts that they didn't quite understand, and for having it to refer to as needed. I made note of this, vowing to reconsider how I present slideshows post-COVID.

While these lectures were visually like what I would present in a face-to-face class, my recorded voice took on a different cadence. I still reviewed materials, told stories, and made parallels between the course content and current events as I would in person, but I found myself speaking softer, slower, and with more ease. I wasn't feeling pressured to "get it all in" before time was up. I was also aware that I was no longer in a room with others where we could pause for questions and engage in spontaneous discord. The time between students viewing the recording and then meeting online for that corresponding lecture seemed to lead to deeper dives, sometimes in verbal discussion and sometimes in just being together without anything to say. Those moments became powerful segues into creating art together in silence. I did not take any lack of verbal discord as suggesting that learning wasn't happening. I trusted the process. I found it affirming that in the end, most students attended all the voluntary meetings and made art.

Social Presence

It was essential for me to be a facilitator and container that was present but not at the centre of attention as I might be if I were standing in front of an in-person classroom. Social presence theory recognizes that unless students' basic needs are met, learning and connecting with one another cannot occur (Whiteside, 2020). Thus, it establishes an essential atmosphere to promote and grow a collaborative community of learners. While not exclusive to andragogy, social presence supports the adult learners' intrinsic motivation to take an active role in their educational experience as well as that of their peers. "Turn and talks" like think-pair-share, small group work, and outside experiences, such as found object walks, field trips, outdoor classrooms, and attending presentations together, help build social presence in face-to-face course delivery. The online "equivalents," such as online discussion boards, random or assigned break-out rooms, webinars, and digitized panel discussions can be effective, but lack impact, when they are not integrated with live, in-person experiences, such as engaging in live practicum experiences and face-to-face meetings with an advisor.

I considered Whiteside's (2020) "classroom as a neighborhood" model for online learning that recognizes self-care, best intentions, recorded "personalized" learning modules, clearly labeled and outlined tasks. This also included multiple avenues for communication, compassion and patience for repeated questions, and letting go of the reliance on mandated, hours-long synchronous online meetings.

Flexibility

Some of the problems I encountered in our art coffeehouse included environmental distractions of both myself and the students, connectivity failures and interruptions, and an awkward discussion flow brought on by individuals' internet bandwidth and the time lag inherent in digital communication. Having unrealistic expectations with students' internet connections or my own was wasted energy. One day, I lost power during class. I was pleased to learn that the students present that day all stayed on for the duration of the synchronous time and made art together.

After pivoting to unplanned online course delivery, I hoped to balance any disruptions in the flow of learning by carefully crafting instructor-guided asynchronous activities. Conrad and Donaldson (2004) acknowledged many benefits of asynchronous learning materials. These include offering more time for reflection, granting room for depth, providing privacy, and allowing students to self-select their prime time to take in new learning and work at their own pace.

Immersive Learning

Besides the course elements discussed above, it was also important for the course to have a primary hands-on experiential component that supported student learning outcomes and that was not ignorant of the online learning platform. The Expressive Therapies Continuum, or ETC (Hinz, 2020; Kagin & Lusebrink, 1978), was central to the learning in this course. Its six components (kinesthetic, sensory, perceptual, affective, cognitive, and symbolic) informed weekly art media explorations, and its four hierarchical levels provided natural scaffolding for each learning module throughout the course.

In re-envisioning delivery of this course, I became influenced by two frameworks (one educational, one arts-based) to develop a combined structure supportive of scaffolded and immersive learning of the ETC. These were the flipped classroom model (Hawks, 2014; Hew & Lo, 2018; Tolks et al., 2016) as well as Miller's (2012) one-canvas process painting.

Educational Framework 1: The Flipped Classroom

The flipped classroom model is also referred to as the inverted classroom model in higher education. It is "a blended learning method in which a self-directed learning phase takes place before the classroom learning phase" (Tolks et al., 2016, p. 3). An example of this includes my description of the pre-recorded slideshow lectures used in the course. The asynchronous aspects of the course are self-directed (aligning with andragogy) and help develop learning and comprehension of the material, noted as lower-order cognitive skills (Tolks et al., 2016). Self-directed learning shifts away from passive learning, where students sit and listen without the ability to navigate the information at a time and pace that resonates with them. Within this self-directed phase, remembering and understanding occur. In contrast, applying, analyzing, evaluating, and creating occur in the synchronous components (Tolks et al., 2016). I would argue that in COVID times, it was important to facilitate an online classroom that also supported applying, analyzing, evaluating, and creating in asynchronous learning activities, and this can be achieved using an arts-based framework, which is a key element in art therapy pedagogy (Leigh, 2020).

Arts-Based Framework 2: Miller's El Duende

The arts-based framework I selected for this course was Miller's (2012) one-canvas process painting. I had taken a weekend workshop of this method many years ago with art therapist Abbe Miller. I was so moved by the process and how reworking and revisioning one canvas over time, while documenting changes with digital photos and written journal entries, afforded me both a container for my chaos and consistency during uncertainty. It was an emergent process where I held no expectations and was receptive to new learning with both open and active curiosity (Unreal, 2019). I was mindful that the nature of the workshop was intentionally different from the focus of the course I was teaching, and that Miller's process, also known as el duende, is often used in clinical supervision models (Miller, 2012) and not a content-focused course like I was teaching. Yet I felt confident in el duende's inherent process of adding, changing, and altering, and that it would align with the scaffolded art exploration that would become an anchor for this course.

Structuring Students' Asynchronous Art Processes

Six weeks of the course centred on a component on the ETC, starting with the bottom of the framework and working our way up the "ladder." To prepare for this, students were introduced to Miller's el Duende process through literature and with an example of my own creative synthesis from one-canvas process painting work. We discussed how the intention for our use of Miller's process would be different than what Miller had intended and would be aligned with the course objectives, such as to practice skills for developing awareness and insight into art processes, materials, and personal symbolic language.

Synchronous and online discussion board posts helped students to begin by curating their materials. A specific community "watercooler" section of BlackBoard was established where students could ask questions about the course and share relevant links and anecdotes with one another. Students were encouraged to stop by the watercooler regularly to help their fellow peers.

Figure 12.1 is a still photograph from a video shared with students of my kinesthetic component exploration (Hinz, 2020) where I demonstrated using what I could resource from my environment. The cardboard became my "canvas" for the duration of the course. Some students used refurbished or upcycled canvas. Others used fabric as a basis (Figure 12.2), and another used digital media in combination with found objects and "traditional" materials which were then imported into the digital realm. As we continued to add and build, or alter and change, with each new ETC component, we stayed in relationship to the original foundation. Like Miller's (2012) process, students documented the stages of change through photographs and written reflection. What we added was a model of sharing and peer and instructor assessment and feedback using video blogging (see the subsection "what's your super-power…?"). At the end of the course, students were instructed to submit a video of their creative synthesis, documenting all phases of the arts process and highlighting each component and level of the ETC framework. A corresponding final integrative paper planned to accompany this project was made optional, which was a decision made collaboratively between the instructor and students, based on current events that were negatively impacting students' overall wellbeing.

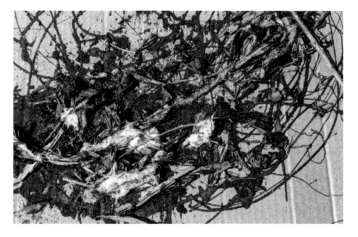

Figure 12.1 Instructor's Kinesthetic Component Exploration

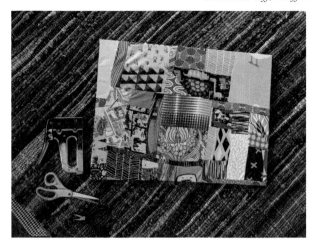

Figure 12.2 Hanna's Stretched Fabric Basis for the ETC El Duende Project

Instructor's Reflection: Being Real

In addition to delivering course content, I used the art coffeehouse to share notes to the class and artwork I created alongside them. What I had hoped would be most helpful for the students was also most helpful for me. I missed seeing the students in person (Figure 12.3). I missed our shared physical spaces (Figure 12.4). I missed being physically present with their energy, the spontaneity of art studio happenings, and the tangents our conversations would wind through when we were together. Therefore, in this section, I have included some of the themes highlighted in correspondences I sent to students.

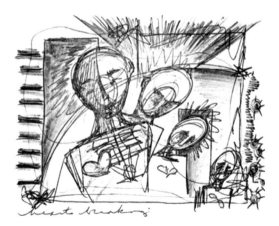

Figure 12.3 Instructor's Drawing—Hearts Breaking

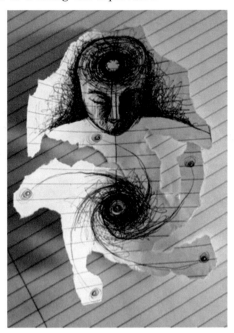

Figure 12.4 Instructor's Drawing—Zoom Drain

Correspondence Through Announcements

My institution's learning management system has an announcement function that is posted on the main page of the course shell and then automatically emailed out to students enrolled in the course. I utilized the announcements function frequently. It was important to "show up" for students throughout the course. Video, voice, text, and art responses provided alternative ways students could receive messages and communication from the instructor, which modelled the communication they would be tasked to do as a part of the course, such as peer assessments. Using announcements in this manner supported both sociological and emotional strands of learning (Dunn et al., 1995) to pave a non-threatening path towards being a community of learners and the peer assessments they would be engaging in. I was not simply the course facilitator; I was also a part of this community of learners. A "guide on the side"; not a "sage on the stage."

What's Your Superpower to Get Through This Quarter?

A pre-course announcement with the prompt "what's your superpower...?" offered a low-stakes practice assignment and introduced the students to Flipgrid, a website and application that allows teachers to create "grids" for video blogging and discussions (https://info.flipgrid.com/). There were practical reasons for choosing Flipgrid, as it does not need to be downloaded, can be used with any camera-enabled device, has security settings that can be customized, and it is free. The instructor can introduce a topic by text, voice, and/or video and set a time limit for the recording of each module or grid. The students took to this platform with ease and performed functions with filters, stickers, GIFs, and other tricks of which I was not even aware.

Alone Together: An Example of an Emergent Correspondence

This example highlights a time I shared an art response with the class (Figure 12.3). During that synchronous class time, which prompted my art response, something felt different, and I acknowledged that while our time together seemed "awkward and clunky: an artificial connection," I felt most connected to them when we fell into silence, making art, alone together.

Silence is a natural occurrence in art therapy (Regev et al., 2016) and sometimes we are not sure if that is a good thing or a bad one. Instead of choosing between the two, I offered the students another option: to simply make observations without judgment. I asked students to recall if they had ever felt the need to fill a silence while working with a client, or if they had ever witnessed a client needing to fill the silence. Then students were prompted with the question, "Have you ever asked the art therapy participants/clients what silence may mean for them?" and it became an emergent reflective assignment for their journal entries. I ended the communication by affirming that we all may have had interpreted the silence in our class time very differently. I disclosed that I could only speak for myself, but that I felt warmth, love, and togetherness as we communicated without words, alone together.

Student Highlight: Hanna Lee

I am grateful for Hanna and her kindness in giving me permission to share her creative synthesis project with readers. The images (Figures 12.5, 12.6, and 12.7) show two details of her project and the final piece. The video Hanna submitted for project completion, set to music, can be viewed here: https://tinyurl.com/HLElDuende.

Hanna did not offer written feedback on the course for this chapter, which is a beautiful affirmation for the message of "cameras off, coffee on." Class participation was not performative. It was about being a part of something meaningful during challenging times, growing our neighbourhood connections through arts-based practices and learning, and being alone together. I did not need to directly *hear* in a formal paper what Hanna had learned. She demonstrated her embodied learning through peer assessments and feedback, through video blogging on Flipgrid about how she integrated course content in arts-based practices, and by exhibiting how she assimilated the vast amount of material through her creative synthesis. While the creative synthesis was not the only way in which I could assess Hanna's learning and growth in this course, it was one way that

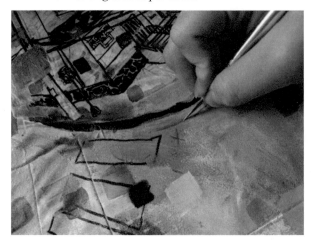

Figure 12.5 Hanna Utilizing the Cognitive Component of the ETC

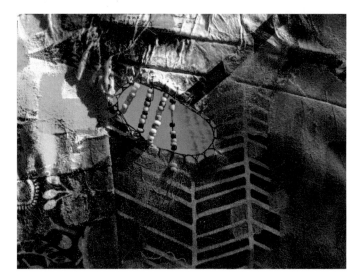

Figure 12.6 Detail of Hanna's Final Piece

complimented all the other areas addressed to support a learner-centred constructivist model, with flexibility, with social presence, and in creating a classroom neighbourhood filled with compassion and care.

Conclusion

Teaching and learning took on new meaning at the onset of the COVID-19 pandemic, specifically for those programs not designed for online course

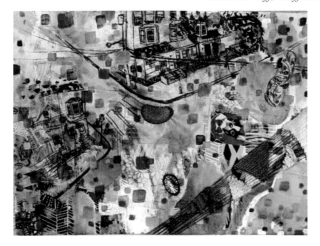

Figure 12.7 Hanna's Creative Synthesis of the ETC El Duende

delivery. As an instructor, I took the shift to online as an opportunity to interrogate my teaching philosophy and take a critical look at the reality of the course load in a pandemic, and how to deconstruct and rebuild a more equitable, compassionate, flexible course that still delivered on its desired learning outcomes. I was brave to do things differently than what was being recommended in response to emergency remote online teaching, such as I diverted from meeting synchronously online just as if the class was meeting in person and requiring cameras to be turned on to monitor participation and attendance.

I became influenced by two frameworks to develop an immersive learning experience of the Expressive Therapies Continuum. Firstly, I followed the flipped classroom model (Hawks, 2014; Hew & Lo, 2018; Tolks et al., 2016) by putting the primary information load on online learning materials that students go through on their own before class time and then use our synchronous class time to ask questions, reflect, and process. Secondly, I applied Miller's (2012) one-canvas process painting approach, which involves the reworking and revisioning of one canvas over time, while documenting changes with digital photos and written journal entries. This enabled for the construction of new learning.

As much as I needed to take the course apart and rebuild it, students were required to forget how they had been taking classes before and discover new ways of learning. Our journey together was sometimes messy but always interesting. We figured it out, and in doing so developed a learning community steeped in collaboration and compassion. Social presence stayed at the core of it. Each time we met, we had our coffee on and our art supplies ready, with the simple intention to be together and spend some time with our classroom neighbours and friends.

Acknowledgements

I would like to thank the students of the Spring 2020 *Creativity, Symbolism, and Metaphor in Art Therapy and Counseling* course, and Hanna Lee for her student leadership and gift of sharing her creative synthesis to showcase the course's learning outcomes. I would also like to thank Drs. Stephen Gambescia, Fran Cornelius, and Dana Kemery for their teachings and guidance in andragogy and online teaching, and my colleague Dr. Natalie Carlton for never doubting me.

References

Brach, T. (2019). *Radical self-compassion: Learning to love yourself and your world with the practice of RAIN*. Viking.

Brookfield, S. D. (1990). Teaching: A complex and compassionate experience. In S. D. Brookfield (Ed.), *The skillful teacher* (pp. 1–19). Jossey-Bass.

Conrad, R., & Donaldson, J. A. (2004). Designing online engagement. In R. Conrad & J. A. Donaldson (Eds.), *Engaging the online learner: Activities and resources for creative instruction* (pp. 16–23). Josey-Bass.

Dennick, R. (2012). Twelve tips for incorporating educational theory into teaching practices. *Medical Teacher, 34*(8), 618–624. https://doi.org/10.3109/0142159X.2012.668244.

Dunn, R., Griggs, S. A., Olson, J., Beasley, M., & Gorman, B. S. (1995). A meta-analytic validation of the Dunn and Dunn model of learning-style preferences. *The Journal of Educational Research, 88*(6), 353–362. https://doi.org/10.1080/00220671.1995.9941181.

Fish, B. J. (2019). Response art in art therapy: Historical and contemporary overview. *Art Therapy, 36*(3), 122–132. https://doi.org/10.1080/07421656.2019.1648915.

Hawks, S. (2014). The flipped classroom: Now or never? *American Association of Nurse Anesthetists Journal, 82*(4), 264–269.

Hew, K. F., & Lo, C. K. (2018). Flipped classroom improves student learning in health professions education: A meta-analysis. *BMC Medical Education, 18*(38), 1–12. https://doi.org/10.1186/s12909-018-1144-z.

Hinz, L. D. (2020). *The expressive therapies continuum: A framework for using art in therapy*. Routledge.

Kagin, S. L., & Lusebrink, V. B. (1978). The expressive therapies continuum. *Art Psychotherapy, 5*(4), 171–180. https://doi.org/10.1016/0090-9092(78)90031-5.

Leigh, H. (2020). Signature pedagogies for art therapy education: A Delphi study. *Art Therapy, 38*(1), 5–12. https://doi.org/10.1080/07421656.2020.1728180.

Miller, A. (2012). Inspired by *el duende*: One-canvas process painting in art therapy supervision. *Art Therapy, 29*(4), 166–173. https://doi.org/10.1080/07421656.2013.730024.

Regev, D., Kurt, H., & Snir, S. (2016). Silence during art therapy: The art therapist's perspective. *International Journal of Art Therapy, 21*(3), 86–94. https://doi.org/10.1080/17454832.2016.1219754.

Taylor, D. C. M., & Hamdy, H. (2013). Adult learning theories: Implications for learning and teaching in medical education: AMEE guide no. 83. *Medical Teacher, 35*(11), e1561–e1572. https://doi.org/10.3109/0142159X.2013.828153.

Tolks, D., Shäfer, C., Raupach, T., Kruse, L., Sarikas, A., Gerhardt-Szép, S., Klauer, G., Lemos, M., Fischer, M. R., Eichner, B., Sostmann, K., & Hege, I. (2016). An introduction to the inverted/flipped classroom model in education and advanced training in medicine and in the healthcare professions. *GMS Journal for Medical Education*, *33*(3), 1–23.

Unreal (2019, March 15). Active curiosity vs. open curiosity [Blog post]. *Lesswrong*. https://www.lesswrong.com/posts/22LAkTNdWv6QaQyZY/active-curiosity-vs-op en-curiosity.

Whiteside, A. (2020, April). Remembering social presence: Higher education remote teaching in COVID-19 times [Blogpost]. Regional Educational Laboratory Program. https://ies.ed.gov/ncee/edlabs/regions/southeast/blog/2020_04_10_remote_teaching.asp .

13 Integrating Art Therapy with Nature-Based Practices

Pamela Whitaker, Nicola Shaw and Michelle Winkel '

Introduction

Wherever you find yourself right now, we encourage you to feel connected to the earth beneath you and know it speaks to a history, to stories of our ancestors long before we graced the same spaces. Sweeney (2002) saw the benefits of interrelating the theories of art therapy with applied ecopsychology and founded the practice of eco art therapy. This integration of art therapy with nature-based practices in outdoor spaces is a modality where clients can work on their own needs first—with, within, and in-between nature. Nature serves as a role model for self-regulation and can bring restoration for our inner psyches, leading to a rebalancing and reconnection with our outer landscapes.

This chapter will explore two ways of applying eco art therapy as an online practice in training programs: (1) A walking studio with an online component as part of MSc. Psychotherapy training at the Belfast School of Art (Ulster University), and (2) immersion in nature as part of the eco art therapy training program hosted by the Canadian International Institute of Art Therapy (CiiAT).

Nature in Art Therapy

Nature, an invisible yet tangible colleague, full of wisdom and awe, provides her 'clinic.' Imagine pine needles on the edges of branches swaying their tips like fingers, or a beautiful iridescent snail shell stumbled upon in a meadow a million miles from shore, eliciting the notion of 'home.' In an intimate collaboration, nature whispers to the client and therapist, "Come and be with me."

Farrelly-Hansen (2001) explored art therapy in partnership with the earth. She questioned the relevance of current Western medical models and their absence of considering the relationship of people to nature. More recent studies have sought to identify the importance of woodland and natural landscapes for mental health (O'Brien, 2005). Globally, this has included the Japanese practice of 'forest bathing,' where walking activities are encouraged in forest environments to reduce blood pressure levels (Park et al., 2010), and 'sit spotting', a practice of sitting in nature without an agenda to restore mindfulness (Jhung, 2020).

DOI: 10.4324/9781003149538-16

Jordan (2009) discussed whether nature could mirror the positive early childhood attachment styles: secure, anxious-preoccupied, dismissive-avoidant, and fearful-avoidant. His essential idea was that clients who had an ambivalent childhood attachment style were also ambivalent to nature and to their own self-care in adulthood. He wondered if this population would benefit from what he called *EcoTherapy*. We, too, as eco art therapists, have observed the power of art making in and with nature to replicate and heal disruptive attachment patterns. For instance, nature is a great example of how to handle awkward climates and seasons. Many clients can still find life in or underneath the strewn seaweed, or the burnt tree trunk, find hope in the lone cactus with its succulent leaves, or are able to process grief with the growth of a sapling. Incorporating these elements, metaphors, or feelings into art, whether through photo, video, drawings, sculptures, enactments, or blogs, inevitably brings healing and regrowth.

According to Jordan and Marshall (2010), nature found a way to show up and become a co-therapist alongside them in their psychotherapy sessions outdoors. Additionally, Shaw has experienced a subtle difference, where the therapist becomes attuned to being a co-therapist alongside nature, who is already present before, during, and after the session. It is almost as if the therapist acts as a conduit for nature and her messages. Even while accepting and trusting nature and one's intuition, it remains paramount that the therapist keeps the inherent therapeutic framework secure, such as by avoiding too much familiarity with the client. The role of the therapist is to keep holding presence and process together and to catch the client being interested and excited with the materials they pass by, to notice which materials are of resonance or repulsion, and to ultimately offer the client the opportunity to play and be playful. One key philosophical aspect to convey in an online eco art therapy program is mirroring therapeutic aspects that participants would gain outdoors, such as *vitality* and *awe*.

Below we describe the walking studio, one example of the intersection between eco psychotherapy and art therapy.

Pamela Whitaker: Walking Studio

The walking studio discussed in this chapter is a collection of walks undertaken by MSc. Psychotherapy students at the Belfast School of Art (Ulster University) with senior citizens in a major American city. The walks take on the form of impromptu studios, which provide the students with a practicum opportunity involving clients who live in a different part of the world. The walking studio involves an online blog in which client participants document their journeys and impressions. Thus, the walks become commentaries, personal signposts, and artistic endeavors. The walking studio blog (Figure 13.1) (thewalkingstudio.wordpress.com) is an archive of variations in walking practice that follow a line of inquiry. It covers the way in which a walk is composed, executed, and made into an art form.

The Walking Studio

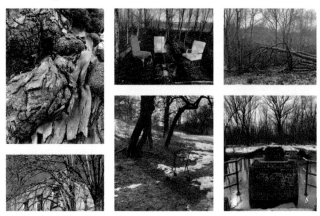

Figure 13.1 The Homepage of the Walking Studio Blog

Walking studios are created by their producers and curators, who design a walk for the experiences found along its route. The artistry of a walk can be generated through words, photographs, sounds, land art, illustrations, assemblages (of found materials), and videos that document happenings along a pathway. The social network of walkers using the methodology of the walking studio bestows a sense of belonging and psychological support. The purpose of a walk, within art therapy, is to find a course of action, one's own path, new routes of exploration, and the making of a personal cartography.

Walking is a marking and a determination to get somewhere (both on the walk and in life). It is also an immersion into our whereabouts, in terms of the social realities of our neighbourhoods, urban environments, and surrounding habitats. The walking studio blog is there for everyone, as a collection of walking experiences and narratives that take each visitor somewhere different in terms of the walkways, scenes, and the themes of each walk. The walk becomes a shared community of practice, where the art media derive from the commonplaces that form a relational conduit in terms of the sharing of experiences (Wenger-Trayner & Wenger-Trayner, 2015).

The art of walking is validated by evidence that suggests it enhances mood, vigor, reasoning, and communication (Cooley, 2021). The artistic release of a walk into the public domain (as a blog post) is an act of dissemination and fortitude. As a form of portraiture and autobiography, a walk can be furthered through its sharing online. The blogging leads to online gatherings and conversations about the walks, creating the sense of taking the walks together, but not at the same time. The viewers are virtual companions who join the experience of the walk after it has been posted online.

Walking as Methodology

Art therapy can encompass the walking studio as a form of public art making and the legacies of mark making that we leave to trace our way. Every walk is a new art form, generated within the locations of a distance travelled. The walking studio blog includes photographs and descriptions that can be reimagined at one's own place and pace so that someone else's walk inspires our next destination.

Walking as a reflective art practice can be documented on a walking app, an art of walking journal, a wayfaring blog, and sound recordings. The walking studio can be represented in photographs that tell stories of what we encounter within and outside ourselves. The term *mobilities*, a method of documentation within the humanities, has been applied to the art of walking, in relation to mobile media practices that capture the features of a walk for others to see (O'Neill & Roberts, 2020). Mobilities is a social paradigm considered to be a form of autoethnography and a performance of space and time. It tracks people's walking narratives and the scenes within which they move. A blog can act like a digital photo book or imaginative journal, depicting the life of a walk as an artistic outcome.

The scenes of a walk are not neutral. Careri (2017) uses the term *transurbance* to describe these vulnerable places that disrupt our equilibriums and ask for our attention, which we may find along walks. The term *transurbance* relates to transgression and walking outside our comfort zones to encounter the realities of civic life that are different from our own. A walk can be an investigation into surroundings that seem wounded and in need of repair, or a connection to people seeking recognition.

The inventiveness of a walk as a studio is its mapping of new territories and productions of subjectivity that take us somewhere different and beyond our personal boundaries of familiarity. The will to deviate is a line of becoming that also exists digitally as an extension of a walk online. Photographs of walks form connections between strangers as a shared resonance and metaphoric referencing to turning points and crossings. Each walk is a transitioning from one place to another, and we are followed (online) by those who wished they had been there, or who want to follow on with their own journey.

A Walk of Life Discussion

The walking studio utilizes a/r/tography (an artistic co-production combining art, research, and teaching) to encourage cooperative knowledge-making, and combined spheres of artistry (Irwin, 2021). It is a methodology that produces both artifacts, such as photographs of the walk, and events that emphasize an adaptation to changing circumstances. It is an approach well suited to walking blog posts that each go somewhere differently, and yet retain an affiliation through a shared platform. The virtual space can bring unique experiences, vicinities, and geographies together. There is a companionship despite physical distances. A/r/tography situates diverse experiences side-by-side as navigation points. Each walk can be approached multiple times within an online community. It exists as both an original reality and, later, reimaged through multiple interpretations. Repeated online visitations make each walk both particular and present for everyone.

A walk may be a symbolic stance, a moving vigil, protest, or pilgrimage (O'Neill & Roberts, 2020). These topics may relate to current affairs, heritage, human geography, politics, contemplation, or a personal quest. The art can also be commemorative as a memorialization of a life event or significant cultural occasion through enactments and ceremony. It is also a relational encounter with people known and unknown, who accompany us virtually and in the actual execution of a walk.

The walking studio is beneficial to art therapy as a creative practice that allows us to fully and physically, with nature, explore and understand others and how they make sense of their worlds. Similarly, the concepts of the outdoor walking studio are at the core of the online eco art psychotherapy course developed at CiiAT, which is discussed in the following section.

Nicola Shaw: An Online Eco Art Therapy Training Program

For clarification, in this section 'Nature' with a capital 'N' is a noun, a tangible entity, a being. The use of writing 'nature' with a small 'n' denotes the outdoor settings, locations and materials. At times, Nature and nature are so intertwined that it is appropriate to author N/nature.

Being immersed outdoors provides a modality through which clients can process a sense of themselves in relation to the world as part of a studio or one-on-one art therapy experience. Initially, CiiAT had conceptualized the Specialised Expressive Arts Training (SEAT) program as a face-to-face intensive eco art therapy training for professional development, but the pandemic necessitated the adaptation of the course for a purely online audience. We translated the essence of the program into six themes: (1) vitality, (2) containment, (3) attuning, (4) integration, (5) honouring, and (6) acceptance. Synthesizing common themes through an a/r/tography approach (Irwin, 2001) was inspired by UK eco psychotherapist Ian Seggins Heginworth (2009), who discovered repetitive themes in his work in correlation with the western months and seasons, such as 'release' in fall.

Authors Shaw and Winkel were the instructors, and chose to keep the class size under ten students because it was a pilot program. All participants, whom we will call trainees in this chapter, had previous mental health training. They also had experience with the videoconference platform Zoom to join us in synchronous class time and the virtual learning platform Moodle to engage with asynchronous teaching elements, such as readings and pre-recorded videos. Furthermore, we watched short training videos synchronously in class, with everyone pressing 'play' at the same time to avoid audio lag, which fostered immediate class discussions. To emulate the processing of transference and countertransference, students and instructors created response art within and after the classes.

Offering a mixture of digital, live classroom sessions and independent home and nature-based play and mock therapy exercises, trainees experienced being a co-therapist with nature. Throughout the program, they attuned themselves to their own preferences, triggers, and biases to locations and materials outdoors. They built confidence, considered ethics, contracts for use with clients, and risk assessments, and experimented with themes and structure in eco art therapy.

Vitality: Environments (or Locations), Thresholds, and Portals

We began the training by celebrating the notion of vitality and awe, of being 'larger than oneself,' through making an art piece in response to this theme. Students introduced themselves by sharing what vitality meant to them, as well as their relationship with N/nature. One trainee described her image (Figure 13.2): "This photo best represents my belief that humans and nature work together, providing reciprocal nurturing and healing" (M. Desjardins, personal communication, 2020).

The use of the digital classroom encouraged trainees to seek out and present photos of their accessible local haunts that they felt were conducive to practicing

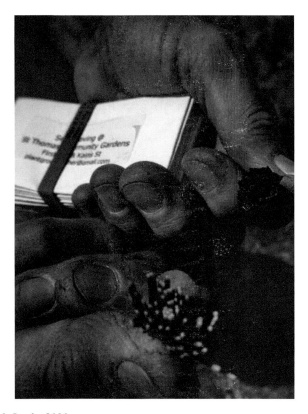

Figure 13.2 Seeds, 2020

this therapeutic modality. One photo depicts a forested stairwell descending into a secluded pool. The wooden stairs became a portal to foster transportation of oneself into a sacred space for therapy. The trainee herself felt awe and wonder in this place. She pondered with us in class if bringing a client to one's own favourite spot in nature was good practice or if it should be reserved for self-care. For another trainee, a simple willow tree could become her new clinic space or studio. Locations such as these could become metaphoric shelters and sanctuaries. As with all training groups, it was essential to recognize and hold this range of emotional states portrayed through the art and photographic responses. The trainees started to empathize with each other, and as practicing professionals, they each played their part in holding the classes as educational training rather than therapy for themselves.

Participants were asked to reflect on the possible themes revealed in each other's favoured locations. Their responses included strength, resiliency, stability, diversity, and regulation. The trainees' creations stirred the essence of vitality and the notion of 'potential' in their hearts and minds during the first training session. With video footage and discussion about suitable outdoor and alternative practice environments, students and teachers emerged with a new curiosity and presence in the digital classroom.

In session one, we specifically addressed the concepts of healthy session openings and closures using portals and thresholds. Akin to an indoor counselling space with walls and a door, in which a client literally enters a 'safe space' and leaves psychological material at the door, creating threshold moments at the beginning and end of sessions becomes a chance in the outdoor environment to do the same. Our training regarding the term 'portals' gives the client (and art therapist) the ability to be transferred into another realm.

The Specialized Expressive Arts Training Program (SEAT) encouraged a site-specific experience after the first class for the trainees to further awaken their senses and a chance to recognize if they need processing due to the vast and rich scope that N/nature provides for stimulation and revitalization. For

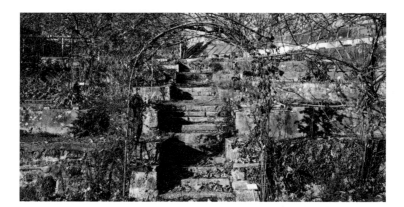

Figure 13.3 A Natural Threshold or Portal

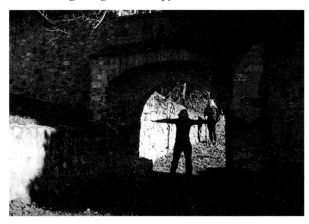

Figure 13.4 An Ancient Monastery Wall Threshold Being Used to Open a Session

some, this might be overwhelming and we invited trainees to complete a 'sense walk' to ground and help manage the extra stimuli. A 'sense walk' is a directive in which one walks or stands for five minutes concentrating on sound, then walks or stands for five minutes concentrating on sight, then follows with touch, smell, and taste (within reason and safety precautions). The online training course provided the platform for uploading images and discussions based on these experiences of reflecting on being static and dynamic with, within, and in-between N/nature. Trainees could notice which senses resonated and which were distracting. This helped them gain understanding into their levels of empathy and patience for the process when working with clients. Journalling afterwards was also recommended.

Containment: Holding the Experiences

As we think about holding sessions outdoors with clients, we explored what kinds of clients might struggle in an outdoor therapy setting by literally 'not having a ceiling.' Class discussions included having to obtain a valid first aid certificate and having basic knowledge of the dangers in outdoor environments related to where one would work, such as weather patterns, steep terrain, poisonous fauna and flora, and protected species. Philosophically, we had conversations about how to respect N/nature (wildlife included) and her resources, including adopting a 'leave no trace' attitude.

As discussed in the previous section, clients would traditionally enter a waiting room and then would enter into an art therapy studio for their session. There would usually be a chance to settle and feel grounded, welcomed, and contained within the walls of the clinic or office space. In eco art therapy, physical boundaries such as ruins, walls, bushes or portals could take on this therapeutic function because the portal provides a threshold for entering. It can contain what was released or brought up during the session.

When artwork is created outdoors, there are often opportunities to incorporate scale and depth that goes beyond what is physically possible indoors. The specific location of artwork and how it is juxtaposed in the landscape can become as important for the client to consider as the work itself. Here, in Figure 13.5, a client extended the shape of a tree trunk to allow himself to sit in safety to write in his journal.

Clients who struggle to define their own boundaries within a vast outdoor space have often appreciated a soft and warm picnic blanket that can be placed on the ground to symbolize a secure base and a tangible presence.

Furthermore, materials like a small amount of sand or flour can be used by clients to create their own boundaries and containment, such as in Figure 13.6. Using an approach of 'mindful photography' to document can help clients to focus, frame, and contain.

We consider it a best practice to have a 'Plan B' for an accessible eco art therapy session, especially due to inclement weather conditions or the deteriorating health of a client. In our virtual classroom, having trainees from around the world on one digital platform helped to broaden the group's thinking regarding the range of potential spaces, such as a greenhouse or willow tree, that would serve eco art therapy. A therapist practicing in rural Canada may consider a shopping mall to be inappropriate, but to a student therapist from urban and densely populated Kuala Lumpur, a fountain in her

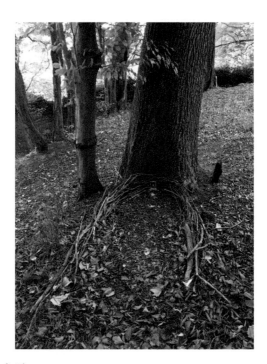

Figure 13.5 Safe Place

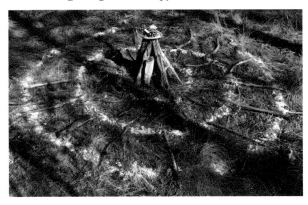

Figure 13.6 Self-Made Containment

local shopping mall was the oasis she could envision for a solid 'Plan B' option. Shaw has fondly reflected how often "being caught out (by weather) is actually being caught in" and precisely what N/nature wants the client to experience and process at that time.

Attunement: Trusting in Presence and Process

There is an array of techniques to ground a client as sessions start, helping them attune to the therapist, their creativity, and to N/nature. At the beginning of a session, we can use singing bowls or empty vessels to centre clients. Additionally, one way of attuning, and becoming fully present into being with N/nature, can be through the aforementioned 'sense walk' or the use of a picnic blanket as an anchor for a secure base.

Immersing oneself in N/ature may have advantages for therapy, as some clients would prefer to not cross the threshold of a clinic or counselling centre. Others may benefit from avoiding the constraints and clinical atmosphere of a therapist's office, where clients may be self-conscious of making a mess with art supplies or making loud noises that disturb people in neighbouring offices. There are no plaques or formal clinical signs on entry into the altered ergonomics of the outdoor art therapy studio. The therapist's guidelines for using the space are more collaborative outdoors, which can contribute to a shift in power dynamics. The idea of accepting and trusting N/nature and one's intuition is pivotal in developing a healthy collaboration between therapist, client, artwork, and nature out in the field.

Being attuned outdoors means noticing all the verbal and non-verbal cues from clients. Language, stance, posture, and gaze are all cues and information to observe about the client's state of health. Noticing if a client has a twinkle in their eye about a certain location or material is an opportunity to invite play and creativity into a session. With shy clients, we might ask if they would like to use a certain material. How is it calling to them to be involved with it, to touch it? Being attuned in the moment as a therapist is key.

Figures 13.7 and 13.8 are taken from an example video that shows how the therapist (in the blue coat) attuned to the client. While out walking, the client spontaneously resonated with the shadow that caught her attention. She was interested in themes of winter and ugliness and was experimenting with the edge of the shadow cast onto the meadow floor. The therapist found herself echoing body movements and gauging distance and proximity to the client to keep containment, awareness, and attachment to the client. The client responded that she felt very supported by the silent engagement of the therapist.

In 1968, Carl Jung noted that there was symbolic power outside under the open sky, being exposed to changing forces (Gomes & Kanner, 1995). This can create a feeling of openness, thus dissipating the insulating effect of the indoor therapy room. Heginworth (2009) expresses that working therapeutically outdoors with a balance of time, space, intent, materials, and privacy is how the

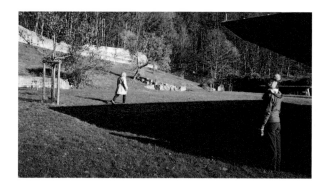

Figure 13.7 Walking the Edge of the Shadow

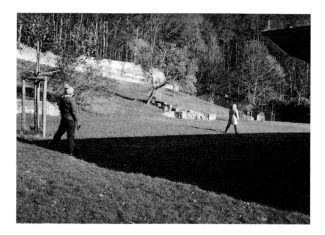

Figure 13.8 Therapist (in Blue Coat) Staying Attached to the Client

client and therapist are able to attune themselves with each other and with the symbolism and metaphors that N/nature and art provide. He often referred to this attunement as 'synchronicity.'

Shaw has witnessed synchronicity during the online training program. For instance, one trainee requested that she wanted the group to watch her in real time working with clay, which she had chosen to represent the nurturing of her inner child. On biodegradable napkins, she had written characteristics that she wanted to honour and folded them into her two pinch pots. Over the screen, there was an air of reverence as she sprinkled sunflower and wild-flower seeds into the pot. We observed her bringing the two halves together and watched as she used her fingers to mold the two halves into one ball. She explained that she intended to go to a local bridge and drop the ball into the river below. She imagined it finding a place, dissolving, and, ultimately, the seeds growing. The collective energy over the digital platform was tangible and meaningful. Staying attuned to these ephemeral moments online can echo the healing moments N/nature provides through synergy and synchronicity.

Integration: With, Within, and In Between

Focusing with, within, and in between N/nature can remind us of how integrated we are to other ecosystems, other biodiversities, and to the 'other' in a spiritual sense. During the SEAT program, a trainee, who wants to be known as Monica, unfolded her story of losing her son. Monica took daily walks with her dog through a woodland, but told us how she was always distracted, her mind focusing on other tasks, because this was where she used to walk together with her son. She had grieved many years ago about her loss, and to Monica, N/nature had lost her sense of tangibility. With the theme of integration and interrelated-ness, we invited trainees to create a visual response to the discussion in the class. In this moment of creation, Monica allowed Nature to enter back into her life.

Monica shared that the tree and this exercise symbolized continuity and a capacity to hold her memories safely. She connected with the idea of *vitality*. She felt *contained* in the space around the sapling, where she found herself remembering and celebrating her son. *Attuning* herself to the moment, she noticed the colors, sounds, textures, and wind weaving movements around the trunk as the softness of the grass held her steady. She felt nature's patience with her. She felt a harmony with her environment and reflected upon the powerful integration of her thoughts and emotions through this whole-body experience. Having the group give their collective attention and gaze was important for Monica and again showed integration, not barriers, of online therapeutic moments.

Honouring: Transference and Countertransference

We have found that honouring nature is not a polite once-off request to tidy any waste away at the end of a session; rather, it is an embedded and some-times spiritual practice of reciprocal respect and dignity, of a continuous and

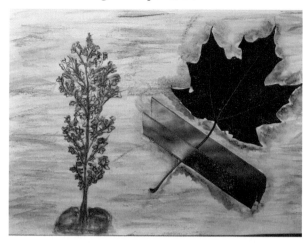

Figure 13.9 'Moments' by Monica

authentic attitude of mindfulness and gratitude. When role modelling this to clients, before long they want to take ownership and begin sessions themselves by offering gratitude to the wildlife and sounds around them, to the strong earth beneath their feet.

Creating a therapist artistic response after each session can help contain the therapeutic process and honour the therapeutic relationship. It facilitates processing clients' stories and helps us empathize with how they see themselves in the world. It is a way for the therapist to continue creating a space to encompass the actions of witnessing and reflecting. In our view, therapist response art is a healthy way of holding the therapeutic frame outside of the session to deal with any residual transference and countertransference.

Shaw writes about her response art, an installation, pictured in Figure 13.10:

> I chose to pick up bulbs off the forest floor and place them into the tree, representing the trainees growing in their own right and gently being placed into the structure of the program. Response art helped me to reveal insights which informed discussions with my co-teacher on modifying our therapeutic training content for the following week, in addition to processing our own countertransference with students' material.

Shaw discovered that creating with natural materials, specifically in the original location of the therapy session, can be a cathartic process, leading to a deeper 'felt sense' (Gendlin, as discussed in Rappaport, 2013), and enabling greater empathy for the client. Gendlin invented the phrase 'felt sense' to describe our inner wisdom that comes through the body in relation to all our experiences in life. Engaging the senses and moving the body to create these installations can add to 'felt sense' or 'embodiment' (Atkins & Snyder, 2018).

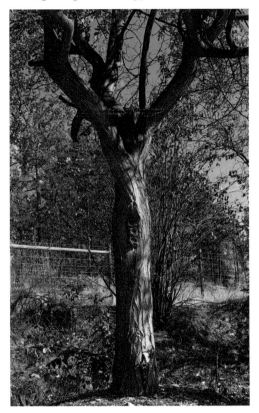

Figure 13.10 SEAT Program Instructor Response Art

Response art gives the time to dwell with content and not to rush (McNiff, 2013). It may reveal to the therapist why a client has juxtaposed certain materials, worked within differing heights and scales, and worked within certain planes. Making response art is a way to honour and synthesize the essence of a session in a live and creative format. When experiencing difficult projections, therapist responses help to transform concerns into manageable metaphors, which can bring relief. The trainees were invited to try this process after one of their mock sessions. One discovered through her installation, created in the original location used for therapy, an honouring towards the reciprocal openness of her mock client to herself as the therapist.

In this program, it was important to consider the shifting dynamics of Schaverien's traditional therapeutic framework model and to consider how transference and countertransference are held within N/nature. Eco therapists have their own framework model labelled the "three-way-relationship" (Berger & McLeod, 2006), connecting the components of client–therapist and nature. With art therapists working within Schaverien's model, what are 'eco' or 'nature-based' art psychotherapists going to use as a guide? Figure 13.11 is

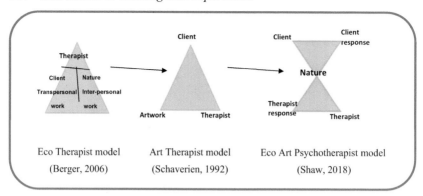

Figure 13.11 Shaw's Eco Art Psychotherapy Model in Context

a new model proposed by Shaw that places nature at the heart of the framework and makes specific reference to include a creative *therapist response* from the art therapist.

With the senses being awakened, a therapist needs to be aware of what triggers them before they work with clients outdoors. Berger (2004) referred to such a triggering, direct encounter with natural elements as 'touching nature-touching the soul.'

Acceptance

During the last SEAT module, trainees shared their experiences by leading mock sessions, which had been their homework for prior weeks. These were sessions with a trusted friend or classmate who had consented to the experience and to support the trainee's learning process and help them encounter the entire continuum of an outdoor session from start to finish. Trainees were required to videotape the sessions, and then, while privately watching the recording of themselves with their client afterward, we asked them to select a short segment that highlighted something special about the session. Later, we screened these video segments in class as a group, watching with each other to provide constructive criticism and share insights and successes. Through Zoom, we navigated a way to witness each student conducting eco art therapy, both in rural and urban places across the globe, with joint focus. One of the main revelations for our trainees was the power of synchronicity occurring through the elements of weather and art materials to reveal their mock clients' emotions. Figure 13.12 demonstrates such a moment with a storm cloud brewing above the mock client's head as she processed family dynamics. The storm began and ended within the creation part of the session!

As the modules came to a close, we acknowledged the unique qualities and the gaps of an online classroom for the tactile and sensorial subject of eco art therapy. Yet, we felt confident that each trainee now had the skills to use N/ nature to enhance their art therapy practice.

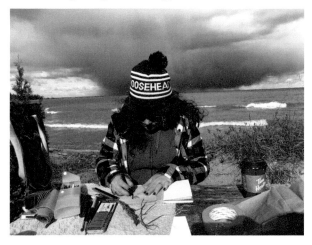

Figure 13.12 Synchronicity through Weather

Conclusion

Being outdoors can provide a much-needed layer of mindfulness to activate the senses and increase the notion of embodiment. Clients may process their understanding and insights about themselves in relation to the world. As a form of expressive studio, a walk outside can stimulate and invite reflection on one's own relationship and purpose in life. This may lead to a creative interaction with the environment, such as the (re)placing of objects or traversing of a path, the framing of the experience in the form of a photograph, or the making of art immersed in the location or elsewhere afterwards, which can then be shared online. As a form of studio, the act of mindfully walking outdoors and creatively engaging with one's surroundings is a feature of eco art therapy and a socially engaged method of being with people. Thus, eco art therapy is adaptive and can be reformulated for experiential learning agendas. It can add to the repertoire of art therapy's capacity as a form of outreach with remote clients of any age.

As this chapter has shown, adding an online component to being in nature provides an effective way to share experiences with other studio participants or classmates. This has the potential to make the individual engagement with nature a lived experience on a broader scale, which is therapeutic for a physical walker as well as those that partake in its narrative virtually, as highlighted by the discussion about the Belfast School of Art walking studio. In the case of the SEAT program, creating a mixture of the digital classroom and homework exercises and videos allowed trainees to experience being a co-therapist with Nature and attune themselves to their own preferences, triggers, and biases to locations and materials outdoors. Redefining frameworks and discussing ethics for outdoor practice were useful for the trainees, who spanned the globe, merging perspectives and philosophies about N/nature in the digital classroom. Following SEAT's six themes, the therapist and client may experience vitality, containment, attuning, integration, honouring, and acceptance as part of a successful eco art therapy practice.

References

Atkins, S. S., & Snyder, M. A. (2018). *Nature-based expressive arts therapy: Integrating the expressive arts and ecotherapy.* London: Jessica Kingsley.

Berger, R. (2004). Therapeutic aspects of nature therapy. *Therapy through the Arts - The Journal of the Israeli Association of Creative and Expressive Therapies, 3,* 60–69.

Berger, R., & McLeod, J. (2006). Incorporating nature into therapy: A framework for practice. *Journal of Systemic Therapies, 25*(2), 80–94. https:/doi.org/10.1521/jsyt. 2006.25.2.80.

Careri, F. (2017). *Walkscapes: Walking as an aesthetic practice.* Ames, IA: Culicidae.

Cooley, S. (2021). Urban walking can be as beneficial as walking in green spaces. https:// samjoecooley.com/2020/04/24/urban-walking-can-be-as-beneficial-as-walks-in-green-spaces/.

Farrelly-Hansen, M. (2001). *Spirituality and art therapy living the connection.* London: J. Kingsley.

Gomes, M., & Kanner, A. (1995). The rape of the well-maidens: Feminist psychology and the environmental crisis. In T. Roszak, M. Gomes, & A. Kanner (Eds.), *Ecopsychology: Restoring the earth healing the mind.* San Francisco: Sierra Club Books.

Heginworth, I. S. (2009). *Environmental arts therapy and the tree of life.* Exeter: Spirits Rest.

Irwin, R. (2021). *A/r/tography: An invitation to think through art-making, researching, teaching and learning.* https://artography.edcp.educ.ubc.ca.

Jordan, M, & Marshall, H. (2010). Taking counselling and psychotherapy outside. Destruction or enrichment of the therapeutic frame? *European Journal of Psychotherapy & Counselling, 12*(4), 345–359. https:/doi.org/10.1080/13642537.2010.530105.

Jordan, M. (2009). Nature and self - an ambivalent attachment? *Ecopsychology, 1*(1), 26–31. https:/doi.org/10.1089/eco.2008.0003.

Jhung, L. (2020). Maximise nature's therapeutic benefits on your next run *Women's Running.* https://www.womensrunning.com/health/wellness/sit-spotting-trail-running/.

McNiff, S. (2013). *Art as research: Opportunities and challenges.* Bristol: Intellect.

O'Brien, L. (2005). *Trees and woodland: Nature's health service.* Farnham: Forest Research.

O'Neill, M., & Roberts, B. (2020). *Walking methods: Research on the move.* London: Routledge.

Park, B. J., Tsunetsugu Y., Kasetani T., Kagawa T., & Miyazaki, Y. (2010). The physiological effects of Shinrin-yoku (taking in the forest atmosphere or forest bathing): evidence from field experiments in 24 forests across Japan. *Environmental Health and Preventive Medicine, 15*(1), 18–26. https:/doi.org/10.1007/s12199-009-0086-9.

Rappaport, L. (2013). Trusting the felt-sense in art-based research. *Journal of Applied Arts and Health 4*(1), 97–104. https:/doi.org/10.1386/jaah.4.1.97_1.

Sweeney, T. (2002). Merging art therapy and applied ecopsychology for enhanced therapeutic benefit. https://www.ecopsychology.org/journal/gatherings6/html/Overview/overview_art_therapy.html.

Wenger-Trayner, E., & Wenger-Trayner, B. (2015). Introduction to communities of practice. https://wenger-trayner.com/introduction-to-communities-of-practice/.

14 Online Art Therapy Classroom in Thailand

Jo Patcharin Sughondhabirom

Introduction

In 2005, when Lucille Proulx (Director Emeritus of the Canadian International Institute of Art Therapy (CiiAT) and The Proulx Global Education & Community Foundation) was volunteering at the Center for Protection of Children's Rights in Bangkok, I was starting a therapeutic arts project with cancer patients in a hospital. As a medical doctor, I often feel the silent sadness in the faces of my patients. In that era, bad news was given to patients in a very brief and direct way. I imagine if the word "cancer" were given to me in such a way, it would probably shut me down and my whole world would collapse. Maybe that was what happened in that silence. Between astonishment and sorrow, the patients could not speak a word. Fixing the communication gap was the very first target of my therapeutic arts project.

In addition, I wanted to widen the use of art therapy in Thailand. This idea brought me to see Lucille Proulx again in 2011. Lucille introduced her colleague, Michelle Winkel, and together we created a formal art therapy training under the term International Program of Art Therapy in Thailand (IPATT) in association with the British Columbia School of Art Therapy, which was later transferred into the hands of CiiAT.

This chapter will discuss the format of the IPATT program before and during the COVID pandemic. A survey will contrast the strengths and weaknesses of online learning as experienced by IPATT students who participated in the program in-person as well as online.

The Format of IPATT Before COVID

The IPATT studio is equipped with audio-visual aids for instructors to present art therapy theories and a studio working area with a wide assortment of art materials that allow students to work experientially. In addition to art therapy education, having students in our studio also gives them opportunities to learn relational literacy inside and outside class time, such as confronting or allying, deepening or skipping, and encouraging or letting go. Inside the classroom, we have students share their ideas or personal stories and the listeners are

DOI: 10.4324/9781003149538-17

offered opportunities to respond. Outside the classroom, we have a tradition that students eat lunch together and some bring their own lunch boxes to share. It is a special moment that we learn about one another and share lessons previously learnt in the classroom. Robbins and Judge (2013) found that when employees from different departments regularly have lunch or coffee together, this deeply affects their behaviour and performance.

The teacher can use sharing opportunities to highlight useful or constructive ways of viewing an event or interpersonal situation (Salmon & Freedman, 2010). In our classroom, when someone starts to share something personal, the instructor often uses the opportunity to demonstrate how to support that person, how to respond to difficult feelings being expressed, and how to close the communication properly. Teaching by modeling is often mentioned as a strength of the program by IPATT students in their end of semester feedback. In supporting students with difficulties, teachers help students bridge the knowledge gained in hypothetical discussions to the real world (Salmon & Freedman, 2010). Furthermore, the more the sharing happens, the more trust is reflected in the relationships (student-to-instructor and student-to-group). Building trusting relationships in the classroom is always our educational goal in addition to the theoretical content and related experiences.

IPATT has carried this in-person format through to the beginning of the year 2020 when the COVID pandemic began and social distancing was mandated.

The COVID Impact on IPATT

Moving the program online entailed changes in how we communicate, the relationships we build, the sharing of intimate stories, and the methods of how we solve problems.

Survey on Five Aspects of Learning

Early in 2021, after three semesters of teaching online, I conducted a small survey with students who experienced both the face-to-face classroom for at least one semester as well as the online classroom for at least one semester (n = 6). All participants were female and had the same instructor in both settings.

This study gauges the effects of the IPATT online teaching program on the quality of the learning compared to our regular in-person classroom experience. Answers were made anonymous by typing them and using post mail services to deliver the answers (rather than emailing), while leaving the sender address blank.

Table 14.1 summarizes the results for the five categories: (a) relationship, (b) communication, (c) support, (d) problem solving, and (e) quality of learning.

In-person, face-to-face teaching received higher scores from the majority of students (4 out of 6) regarding the quality of the relationship between students and instructor. Similarly, 4 out of 6 students perceive the instructor to be quicker in detecting and responding to sensitive issues in face-to-face classes.

Table 14.1 Quality of In-Person vs Online Course Delivery for (N = 6) Participants

		Number of students (out of a total of 6) for whom:		
Main quality categories	Sub categories	In-person classes score higher	In-person and online classes are equal	Online classes score higher
Relationship	Feeling closer	4	2	0
	Feeling confident	3	3	0
Communication	With instructor	2	4	0
	Among group	4	2	0
Support	From instructor (amount)	2	4	0
	Instructor sensitivity	4	2	0
	From student group	3	3	0
Problem solving		1	5	0
Learning		1	5	0

Moreover, communication within the peer group of students was considered more effective by the majority of students (4 out of 6). One explanation for this was that there seemed to be subgroups happening in the online classroom which had shaken the sense of trust among members and thus affected the quality of peer communication. In contrast, the other quality aspects show that at least half, if not more, of the students considered in-person and online class delivery to be equal. Interestingly, no one preferred online classes for any of the learning aspects. As Keret-Karavani & Rolnick (2020) state, "people will not give up the experience of sitting together so quickly" (p. 261).

Since sharing plays a big role in our classroom, we discuss the differences in sharing in an online classroom and sharing in a physical classroom. This discussion is supported by the responses from the student survey.

Advantages of Sharing Online

Detailed survey responses showed that some students felt more comfortable sharing personal stories in the group when they were in their own space, behind the screen, than when they were together in a physical space. They explained that the online classroom offered a certain distance, creating a greater sense of safety. Some felt more comfortable when talking to the camera as opposed to talking in front of a group of people; there was less confrontation in the online setting and the amount of self-exposure seemed under their control. During delicate moments, online classes offered possibilities to hide their vulnerability. With only one click, students could turn off the camera and no one would be able to see them crying. In contrast, about half of the students felt secure in sharing their stories with the group regardless of whether the environment was online or in a regular classroom. One student felt less secure and less comfortable sharing with the online group because they had difficulties judging on screen who they could trust.

My observation is that since the videoconferencing systems place everybody in a visual cell, it emphasizes the separateness of the individuals. The videoconferencing software that we used enlarged the video of whoever was speaking at the time, thereby helping to bring the person forward. Thus, the experience felt closer to an individual encounter and enhanced personal sharing. Keret-Karavani and Rolnick (2020) discuss a similar situation in their chapter about taking space in an online organizational consultancy. The authors wrote that when each participant, including the meeting leader, sits independently in front of the screen,

> this flattened the image of the organizational structure, blurring the visibility of power relation and hierarchy. It allows space for each participant, concretely: to see and be seen, hear and be heard, and symbolically: everyone has his own place and representation on the screen.
>
> (Keret-Karavani & Rolnick, 2020, p. 260)

An additional advantage of the online classroom is that the software prevented the snatching of an individual's turn since it only allowed one person to speak at a time. Students learned to wait for the others to finish. Sharing time became efficient since students were aware of the number of students on the screen and were conscious of what was being shared when it was their turn. This may be different in a face-to-face classroom where the atmosphere and the dynamic of the group influences the mood and tone of the students. This observation suggests that, with a good strategy, deep sharing can happen more in an online setting despite occurring in a conscious stage of mind and is therefore less spontaneous. The cultural aspect comes into play here in societies that have to maintain a behaviour protocol when someone is in a group. In Thai culture, for example, students seem to respond in a more meaningful and openly emotional manner when they are working in their own space.

Another aspect I would like to discuss is the familiarity with new technology. Keret-Karavani and Rolnick (2020) stated that "technology is one more factor that shapes the experience of the session and can affect its results" (p. 258). At IPATT, we found that some students were more keen on technology and electronic devices than others. They were capable of finding solutions when the class encountered technical problems in an online classroom. This offered them opportunities to be considered competent by both themselves and their class. Our instructors often use these opportunities to promote self-esteem in the student(s) and encourage more of this role. This makes it obvious that the online classroom is a co-creation from the beginning, rather than a traditional classroom where the instructor has control of the setting. Keret-Karavani and Rolnick (2020) added that "videoconference medium changes the perception of phenomena known from a co-located meeting, sometimes more salient and other times subtler" (p. 258).

As videoconferencing can pull the speaker forward into full screen, it brings them face-to-face with the audience. In that moment, the speaker's voice is clearly heard; the expression on the face is clearly seen. When the speaker stays very close to the camera, we notice how alert or tired the eyes appear. This kind of information can be a clue that leads to something insightful. One example of this information being useful is from a student in my recent online art therapy classroom. One morning when we were online, it was her turn to present her art piece and the videoconferencing program automatically enlarged her camera feed. While she enthusiastically talked about her art, she briefly mentioned her doubt regarding the artwork's quality before quickly moving on to talk about other aspects of the piece. Even though she spoke in a very low voice, I had a feeling that the student had more to say, but for the moment she decided to pause and refrain. While her mouth was describing the artwork, her eyes were free to roam. As I watched her enlarged, live video stream, I noticed that her eyes were not with the story she talked about. They appeared a little lost. Once she finished, I expressed my admiration for the good work she had done and then asked how life was. The student burst into tears. She had just lost her grandma a few days before the class. The student was functioning as the core of the family, organizing the funeral and hosting the event. In addition, she had to give extra support to her long-time depressed father and was very cautious because of his suicidal history. As a result, the student could not afford to give herself time to feel anything. Her mind was very busy with these many responsibilities. That explained why her eyes appeared to be elsewhere. In a traditional setting, I may have easily missed it because I do not have that audio device in my ears and do not have such close proximity to notice the appearance in her eyes. Weinberg and Rolnick (2020) also noted in their book that "facial expression becomes clearer and in higher resolution online—perhaps even more than in treatment in the same room" (p. 3).

Despite these advantages, there are also disadvantages when sharing online, which I will discuss in the following section.

Disadvantages of Sharing Online

In the online classroom, individualism is exaggerated from the beginning by the fact that each student remains in their own environment and joins the group only through camera. When presenting online, the speaker becomes less conscious of the group as their own image is displayed large on the screen. The audience, seeing themselves and the other group members in separate windows, are visually more aware of the group and yet may still feel isolated. The physical space is not available to inhabit with group members. Thus, group formation was slower in the online classroom. Robbins and Judge (2013) wrote about forming international teams in a virtual world: "it's easy to misinterpret messages without cues like facial expression and tone of voice.

These problems can be even more pronounced among individuals with different cultural backgrounds" (p. 291).

Slow group formation can be explained by the lack of key factors. Although the group members shared a common task in accomplishing learning goals, the separateness in the online format did not support them to feel like a group. The five teaching aspects survey showed that more students felt closer to other group members in face-to-face classes than online. This is likely to be a result of incomplete group formation. I believe it is important to find better ways to form a group through the camera. Creativity of class organizers and instructors may help speed up the process of group formation.

Another disadvantage of online communication is conversing through the video camera. In traditional settings, we naturally look into the eyes of our partner and say what we want to say. By doing this, the person we speak to will notice that the attention is directed towards them. Being the focus of attention, the person is expected to respond. The eye contact connects the two conversing partners together and allows the conversation to go deeper. However, this can be confusing in an online classroom. A student reflected in the survey that, being online with the group, she sometimes did not know where the attention was directed. The eye contact seen on screen was not specific. Being online, so as to connect with the conversation partner, the eyes must aim at the camera, rather than looking into the eyes of our partner in their small window, the position of which has been randomly selected by the program. When responding to what has been shared, the responder must have the sharer in mind and feel what they want to say, but they must also be looking at the camera and say it as if the camera was the person. This is unnatural and requires training.

Lastly, the online software used in our classroom offers the function that we can chat with anyone in the group through text. We can choose to send messages to everyone or to specific members, and it can be done in parallel with the teaching. From personal experience, students used this function to communicate privately with the instructor. For example, when the conversation was getting too emotional, the person would send a small note to me via chat saying that she would be absent from the screen and would turn the camera off. Sometimes they would ask for a more extensive answer through the chat box and let me decide if I wanted to answer in class or to her personally. The tricky part is that this function can be distracting and can promote subgrouping among group members. The fact that we do not know who is exchanging messages in the chat can shake the trusting relationship. Perhaps in the future we find creative ways of using this chat function for creative learning.

Conclusion

The student survey that contrasted in-person and online classroom experiences revealed that face-to-face teaching gets a higher score in 3 out of 9 quality sub-categories; however, most aspects remain the same in both classroom settings. There are advantages and disadvantages to sharing art and personal experiences online, where group dynamics can be different, benefiting some group members but not others. While there is a preference for face-to-face education, the small student survey shows that most IPATT students accept online education as an alternative. We will keep working on improving the quality of learning experience and on cultivating an interest in basic human relationship despite the rapid changes in the virtual world.

References

Keret-Karavani, R., & Rolnick, A. (2020). Practical considerations for online organizational consultancy. In H. Weinberg and A. Rolnick (Eds.), *Theory and practice of online therapy: Internet-delivered interventions for individuals, groups, families, and organizations* (pp. 258–267). Routledge.

Robbins, S., & Judge, T. (2013). *Organizational Behavior* (15th ed.). Pearson.

Salmon, D., & Freedman, R. A. (2010). *Facilitating interpersonal Relationships in the Classroom: The Relational Literacy Curriculum* (1st ed.). Routledge.

Weinberg, H., & Rolnick, A. (2020). Introduction. In H. Weinberg & A. Rolnick (Eds.), *Theory and practice of online therapy: Internet-delivered interventions for individuals, groups, families, and organizations* (pp. 1–10). Routledge.

15 Reducing Anxiety Levels During a Pandemic with Virtual Art Therapy

A Quasi-Experimental Pilot Study

Hedaya AlDaleel, Haley Toll, Michelle Winkel and Christel Bodenbender

Introduction

The COVID-19 pandemic brought an increased need for mental health support. Art therapists, like other mental health providers, made rapid decisions to transition from in-person to virtual formats (Miller & McDonald, 2020; Potash et al., 2020). The Canadian International Institute of Art Therapy (CiiAT) in Victoria, Canada, provides online diploma and certificate programs in art therapy with a requirement for practice in settings, such as hospitals and community organizations. Due to contact restrictions in early 2020, the non-profit Proulx Global Education and Community Foundation, which oversees CiiAT, set up a Virtual Art Therapy Clinic (VATC) to meet the needs of practicum students and serve clients dealing with anxiety and other challenges. Students could continue with their practicum while providing accessible and affordable art therapy services to clients at home. VATC uses the Jane Application (Jane Software Inc., 2020a) as its video conferencing and scheduling platform, which is privacy compliant following Canadian regulations (PIPEDA). Clients can virtually receive art therapy services from VATC anywhere globally by setting up appointments with supervised CiiAT student art therapists.

In this chapter, we describe a CiiAT student-initiated pilot quantitative research study in which student art therapists recorded their clients' anxiety levels before and after virtual art therapy sessions. Preliminary findings suggest that remote art therapy sessions may be a suitable treatment modality for anxiety, particularly during the current global COVID-19 pandemic.

Art Therapy and Experiences of Anxiety

Four years before the COVID-19 pandemic, the World Health Organization reported that one in five people experience depression or anxiety (Brunier, 2016). A Canadian poll conducted in 2018 found that 41% of Canadians reported experiencing anxiety, and about one-third have an anxiety disorder diagnosis and/or are taking antidepressants to treat anxiety (Kirkey, 2018). Anxiety disorders involve fear as a response to a real or supposed somatic or environmental threat. They are physically associated with muscle tension and

DOI: 10.4324/9781003149538-18

vigilance to prepare for future danger and can present as cautious or avoidant behaviours (American Psychiatric Association, 2013). Types of anxiety disorders can include generalized anxiety disorder, panic disorder, and phobia-related disorders (National Institute of Mental Health, 2018, para. 2). Treatments for anxiety depend on the individual's preference, access to mental health care (including insurance), and the type of anxiety disorder diagnosed.

In the practice of art therapy, [a]rt making (such as painting, drawing, sculpting, clay modelling) "is seen as an opportunity to express oneself imaginatively, authentically, and spontaneously, an experience that, over time, can lead to personal fulfillment, emotional reparation, and transformation" (Malchiodi, 2007, p. 6). Psychological distancing of oneself from an emotion while creating art may improve cognitive regulation of emotions by developing meta-cognitive understandings of experiences, such as thinking about our thinking processes (Abbing et al., 2019). For example, during the creative process, the creator can experience a feeling of being in control, which can counterbalance overwhelming emotions inherent in the experience of anxiety (Abbing et al., 2019). In addition, the visual, sensory, and non-verbal aspects of art therapy can be suitable for individuals with anxiety who have difficulty cognitively labelling or naming their emotions (Abbing et al., 2019).

Neurobiologists and trauma specialists propose that traumatic memories and emotional experiences are remembered and felt in the body through three senses. These include exteroceptive senses of phenomena outside of the body (such as sight, smell, taste, touch, taste, etc.), interoceptive senses inside the body (such as pain, kinesthetic movement, cold, hunger, etc.), and proprioceptive senses within the body (such as sense of force, heaviness, limb position and movement, "gut feelings," etc.) (Czamanski-Cohen & Weihs, 2016; Hass-Cohen & Findlay, 2015; Malchiodi, 2017; Sherrington, 1906; van der Kolk, 2014). These bodily sensations and emotional experiences can be challenging to express cognitively and logically with words. Nonetheless, through artistic symbols, metaphors, and movement during the process of art making, individuals can express these experiences that words may not capture (Dew et al., 2018; Malchiodi, 2017). In addition, art making can help individuals self-regulate and relax their body's fight, flight, or freeze system, which is often elevated when experiencing anxiety and stress (Malchiodi, 2017). This can be done through physical art making that incites self-soothing behaviours, such as hand-stitching sculptures with soft fabric or painting soothing landscapes in watercolour to soft music.

Various studies have assessed the ability of art therapy sessions or artmaking to decrease anxiety in diverse individuals, including women (Abbing et al., 2019), healthcare workers (Visnola et al., 2010), undergraduate students (Sandmire et al., 2012), medical inpatients (Shella, 2018), and patients experiencing psychiatric diagnoses (Chambala, 2008). For example, a randomized controlled trial in the Netherlands found that 10 to 12 sessions of art therapy significantly decreased anxiety symptoms and improved 59 clients' subjective reports of quality of life versus a control group (Abbing et al., 2019). Other research studies have found that art making (Curry & Kasser, 2005; Kaimal et al., 2016) and art therapy reduced cortisol levels, which is a biomarker that indicates high levels of stress in the body (Visnola et al., 2010; Kaimal et al., 2017; Laurer & van der Vennet, 2015).

Anxiety During the COVID-19 Pandemic in Canada: A Case for Virtual Art Therapy

Human history recounts various trying moments, including previous pandemics, economic crises, and genocides. Nonetheless, COVID-19 is unique because of its large-scale media attention and a long-term, global lockdown to reduce contagion (Kendall-Tackett, 2020), such as the containment measures recommended by the World Health Organization (2020a). In Canada, these recommendations and research findings have influenced federal and provincial emergency lockdowns and physical distancing measures (Government of Canada, 2020). This drastic change in living, sense of safety, and socializing has affected people physically, emotionally, psychologically, and spiritually. Nonetheless, the full extent of the repercussions of the pandemic are still unknown.

In an opening paragraph of a policy brief, The World Health Organization (2020b) states that "[a]lthough the COVID-19 crisis is, in the first instance, a physical health crisis, it has the seeds of a major mental health crisis as well, if action is not taken" (p. 2). Currently, governments are monitoring the impact of the COVID-19 pandemic on mental health, such as in China (Bao et al., 2020) and Canada (Statistics Canada, 2020). For example, in China, Wang et al. (2020) conducted an online study to measure anxiety, depression, and stress. Furthermore, Xiao et al. (2020) conducted a cross-sectional observational study to ascertain "the effects of social support on sleep quality and function of medical staff who treated patients with COVID-19" (p. 1). These authors have found that diverse populations' mental health worsened during the COVID-19 pandemic due to increased psychological and emotional distress (Rajkumar, 2020; Statistics Canada, 2020). In a recent literature review of 28 articles, Rajkumar (2020) found that rates of anxiety and depression (16–18%) and felt experiences of stress (8%) increased.

In Canada, where 75% of our study participants reside, the federal government studied the extent of psychological distress with an online survey conducted during the first wave of the pandemic, from April 24 to May 11, 2020. Approximately 46,000 Canadians participated, with 88% reporting that they experienced at least one symptom of anxiety related to COVID-19 in the two weeks prior to completing the survey (Statistics Canada, 2020). Anxiety was measured using the Generalized Anxiety Disorder 7-item scale (Spitzer et al., 2006), which is frequently used in anxiety-related population health studies (Statistics Canada, 2020). The study found that "[f]eeling nervous, anxious or on edge" was the most reported symptom (71%), followed by "becoming easily annoyed or irritable" (69%) and "trouble relaxing" (64%) (Statistics Canada, 2020, p. 3). Among those who reported that their mental health worsened since physical distancing began, 41% of respondents reported symptoms consistent with moderate or severe anxiety.

An online survey of 2,761 Canadian adults by Mental Health Research Canada, published in December 2020, also found an increase in reported anxiety (23%) and depression (15%) levels compared to the first pandemic wave that was polled in April 2020. The authors found that "the proportion of Canadians reporting high levels of anxiety quadrupled while depression doubled following the start of the outbreak" (Mental Health Research Canada, 2020, p. 5). Primary COVID-19-related concerns identified include social isolation, fears about family members becoming infected with COVID-19, as well as anxieties surrounding job loss and the economic downturn. The COVID-19 pandemic has deeply affected the mental health of Canadians and others. The World Health Organization (2020b) recommended that nations "[e]nsure widespread availability of emergency mental health and psychosocial support" (p. 3).

Virtual Art Therapy to Treat Anxiety

Providing art therapy via telecommunication technologies can help mental health providers support clients safely during social distancing measures, such as during an international pandemic (Miller & McDonald, 2020). Online accessibility can thus, ultimately, increase participation of people who may otherwise not be able to access therapy services in-person. Videoconferencing as a means for teletherapy has been used effectively by psychotherapists, psychologists, therapists, and mental health providers to deliver services since the 1990s (Berryhill et al., 2019). In a systematic review of videoconferencing psychotherapy for anxiety disorders, Berryhill et al. (2019, p. 54) found the following advantages of providing mental health services through video conferencing: lower cost; high patient satisfaction; accessibility for individuals in rural locations; addressing stigma limitations; accessibility for patients with agoraphobia who prefer to not leave their homes. Furthermore, Berryhill et al. (2019) noted that quality of care in videoconferencing can be equivalent to face-to-face interventions.

Ethnographer Howlett (2021) believes that digital technologies and the restrictions due to the global pandemic are blurring the lines between private, personal, and international boundaries. This affects how people conceptualize temporal space and online relationships (including therapeutic relationships) with wider use of new technologies. Jones et al. (2018) found that the nature of communicating through technology created a unique dimension to a group of female cancer patients as power dynamics became less hierarchical. They observed that "communication via the technology was not necessarily a poor relation to its face-to-face counterpart" (p. 313).

Art therapy via videoconferencing is an emerging practice (Jones, 2017; Walls, 2018), although some innovative researchers, such as Collie & Čubranić (1999), have been writing about distance delivery of art therapy, such as via telephone, online chat forums, discussion boards, and email, for decades. Practice-based research about virtual online art therapy has been conducted with rural veterans (Levy et al., 2018), adolescents with anorexia nervosa (Shaw, 2020), and people who are displaced due to geopolitical conflicts (Usiskin & Lloyd, 2020).

Developing nuanced and accessible art psychotherapy practice and theory must be considered with clients' needs and safety in mind (Shaw, 2020). Discussions about ethical considerations for providing virtual art therapy through videoconferencing have been explored by art therapists Malchiodi (2018) and Walls (2018). As American authors, the ethical recommendations are influenced by the American Psychological Association Guidelines (Joint Task Force for the Development of Telepsychology Guidelines for Psychologists, 2013; Malchiodi, 2018; Walls, 2018). For example, art therapists must consider their expertise with using telecommunication technology to help clients, maintain security and confidentiality when storing and transmitting data, and apply multicultural competence, among other considerations (Malchiodi, 2018; Walls, 2018). Various art therapists (Malchiodi, 2018; Usiskin & Lloyd, 2020; Walls, 2018) recommend that art therapists consider the "digital divide", including generational and economic differences regarding accessibility and comfort in using digital technology when considering this form of therapy. The authors thus recommend that art therapists interested in using virtual platforms to deliver therapy make attempts to reduce inequitable barriers. Therefore, research that attempts to understand clients' experiences of virtual art therapy is needed, particularly in a practicum training program with art therapist students.

Research Design: The Virtual Art Therapy Clinic

This quasi-experimental pre-post study examines the use of virtual individual art therapy for the alleviation of anxiety of 87 adult clients (over 18 years of age). These individuals have chosen to participate in individual sessions with student art therapists in the Virtual Art Therapy Clinic. The quantitative pilot study utilizes information collected by 15 student art therapists who had completed several core art therapy foundation courses, had training in conducting intakes and art therapy online, and were guided by registered supervisors. The students facilitated a total of 774 virtual art therapy sessions through the VATC. This research study was approved by the Ethics Committee of the Canadian International Institute of Art Therapy and is ongoing. Findings presented here are based on the first year of data collection from May 16, 2020 to May 15, 2021.

Quasi-Experimental Study in Health Research

The quantitative quasi-experimental study design was chosen because it allows for an investigation of non-randomized therapeutic interventions. This research design is often chosen when it is not feasible or ethical to conduct a randomized controlled trial, as all clients seeking virtual art therapy services need immediate treatment and support (Harris et al., 2006). Sometimes called pre-post-test interventions, quasi-experimental studies are employed to evaluate the benefits of specific treatments (Bennett et al., 2020). The increasing capacity of healthcare institutions to collect routine clinical data has led to the growing use of quasi-experimental study designs in the field of medical informatics as well as in other medical disciplines (Harris et al., 2006). For art therapy, in particular, "a practitioner can't withhold art therapy treatment from a vulnerable group of clients just for the sake of comparison" (Kapitan, 2018, p. 71), which explains the absence of a control group.

Administration of the Assessment

During the 12 months of this study, student art therapists used three Likert 10-point scale questions to measure changes in their clients' anxiety levels before and after virtual art therapy sessions. Student art therapists 'shared' their computer screen with their clients to complete the Likert scale questions online and recorded the scores directly into the clients' confidential online charts. The 3-question Likert 10-point scale (see section Anxiety Scoring Method on p. 200) was used before and after every virtual art therapy session and was administered verbally. The student art therapists recorded scores for each session in Jane, a telehealth platform, as they shared the content of their screen with the client. Each student art therapist indicated their client's score by dragging the slider to the number that the client expressed on a scale of 1 to 10 for each of the 3 questions. Therefore, anxiety levels were measured consistently throughout sessions and over time. Sessions in which all three anxiety scores were not recorded were eliminated from the study. This resulted in 774 sessions with a complete set of 3 data points, which became the basis of this study. Clients signed a consent form for virtual art therapy, as well as participation in the research project. The data was stored confidentially in Jane.

Participants

Participants voluntarily booked sessions with 1 of our 15 student art therapists through the web-based clinic at the following website: https://arttherapy.network/ (Proulx Global Education and Community Foundation, 2021). Only participants above the age of 18 were included in this study. To protect client privacy, in accordance with Walls' (2018) online art therapy recommendations, digital codes were used as identifiers for data collection and analysis. Consent was obtained in the first session when the art therapist discussed the built-in intake form and the consent clauses with the client by screen share, and the client signed the form. Table 15.1 provides an overview of the stated gender, geographic location, and average age of the clients that participated in this research. Of the 87 participants, 61 live in Canada, which makes Canadians the largest participant group (70%).

Table 15.1 Participant Demographics

Number of client participants	87
Average age (years)	39
Self-identified gender	
Female	78
Male	6
Non-binary	3
Geographic distribution	
Canada	61
USA	13
Egypt	4
Great Britain	3
Thailand	2
India	1
Brazil	1
Saudi Arabia	1
Sweden	1

Virtual Art Therapy Platform

The Jane Application (Jane Software Inc., 2020a) was selected as the video conferencing portal and data storage for the VATC. Jane was chosen because it is the product of a Canadian company with headquarters in British Columbia, which aided accessibility to technical support during the early setup phases. The browser-based software required no installation of additional software for clients and was affordable for the non-profit foundation.

Jane provides online booking, charting, scheduling, secure videoconferencing, and invoicing on one secure system (Jane Software Inc., 2020a). This platform is compliant with the Canadian Personal Information Protection and Electronic Documents Act (PIPEDA) (Jane Software Inc., 2020b). Therefore, all information entered in Jane is safely and securely stored, according to the privacy laws applied in Canada.

Anxiety Scoring Method

We developed the *CiiAT Anxiety Likert Scale* (CALS) to score differences in anxiety levels from the beginning of the session to the end and also from past week to the end of the session. Likert scales are considered a reliable method for obtaining qualitative data on a population, such as in the 4-question-based Outcome Rating Scale (Bringhurst et al., 2006) or the 10-item Patient Psychotherapy Process Scale (Carter et al., 2011). With the Likert scale, clients can intuitively identify their current emotional state on a given range continuum. Past anxiety research (Davey et al., 2007) has utilized similar Likert scales with few items and shown their reliability. Additionally, "brief outcome assessment measures have obvious face validity and meet the minimal criteria of psychometric adequacy" (Campbell & Hemsley, 2009, p. 2). The CALS was developed because it was simple and quick to administer and, thus, feasible for use in each session without taking too much time away from art therapy.

The CALS assesses self-reported feelings on a scale of one to ten; ten signifies extremely anxious, while zero signifies no anxiety. Student art therapists asked clients the following questions before and after the virtual art therapy sessions:

1   On a scale of 0–10, how anxious do you feel right now before the session?
2   On a scale of 0–10, how would you rate your anxiety over the week?
3   On a scale of 0–10, how anxious do you feel now after the session?

Questions (1) and (2) were asked at the beginning of the session, whereas question (3) was asked at the end. Thus, the CALS allows us to measure:

- The difference in anxiety between the past week and the beginning of the session. What is the therapeutic effect of simply going to get help?
- The difference in anxiety between the beginning of the session and the end of the session. How much did the session help the client alleviate the anxiety they reported feeling at the beginning?
- The difference in anxiety between the past week and at the end of the session. How much did the session help the client alleviate the anxiety they reported feeling over the preceding week?

Scores were taken from the client charts in Jane and entered into a spreadsheet for each client and each session, which allowed us to apply calculations for mean, median, standard deviation, variance, and t-test over the data points of all client sessions that were included in this study.

Results

The CALS was used to determine whether attending 60-minute virtual art therapy sessions with student art therapists alleviated anxiety for 87 adult clients. Anxiety data was collected by the student art therapists for 774 client sessions over the span of 12 months. CALS questions (1) and (2) were asked at the beginning of each client session, whereas item (3) was asked at the end. Table 15.2 and Table 15.3 display and compare the CALS results.

In a series of interviews, student therapists reported that they were comfortable and confident transitioning from in-person to virtual art therapy sessions. They felt supported by the clinic administrative team and were grateful for the opportunity to continue accumulating their practicum hours. Some of the student therapists found it challenging to remember the CALS questions each time,

Table 15.2 CiiAT Anxiety Likert Scale (CALS) Scores over 12 Months for (N = 87) Participants

Timing of Assessment	Question Posed	Reported Anxiety levels			
		Mean	Median	Standard Deviation	Variance
Beginning of Session	1. On a scale of 0–10, how anxious do you feel right now before the session?	4.62	5	2.45	6.0
Over past week	2. On a scale of 0–10, how would you rate your anxiety over the week?	5.37	5	2.33	5.43
At session end	3. On a scale of 0–10, how anxious do you feel now after the session?	2.97	3	2.15	4.62

Table 15.3 Comparing Mean CiiAT Anxiety Likert Scale (CALS) Scores (N=87) and Statistical Significance

Comparisons between Client-reported Mean Anxiety Levels	Reduction in Mean Anxiety Scores	Reduction in Mean Anxiety Scores as a Percentage	t Stat	P (T<= t) one tail
Average reported level of anxiety over past week vs. beginning of art therapy session	0.75 (= 5.37–4.62)	14%	t = 10.18	p < 0.0005
Average reported level of anxiety during the start of session vs. end of art therapy session	1.65 (= 4.62–2.97)	36%	t = 28.86	p < 0.0005
Average reported level of anxiety over past week vs. end of art therapy session	2.40 (= 5.37–2.97)	45%	t = 24.75	p < 0.0005

Note. Levels of anxiety were rated on an Anxiety Likert Scale (CALS) scores, from 0–10, over 12 months with a total of 87 participant clients. Questions were posed to participants by student art therapists. The means of the scores are presented in this table.
P-Values for One-Tailed Paired T-Test (Alpha = 0.05; Degrees of Freedom df = 773)

especially when the client came to therapy with needs unrelated to anxiety. Most, however, liked the CALS as a marker that informed them about the needs of the client and the effectiveness of the intervention.

Table 15.3 displays when anxiety was reduced by comparing clients' average reported anxiety levels before, after, and during the week (retrospective).

Participants show the greatest reduction in anxiety (2.4) when comparing the reported anxiety levels from over the past week (5.37 out of 10) to the anxiety levels at the end of the art therapy session (2.97 out of 10). When comparing average self-reported levels of anxiety between the beginning (4.62 out of 10) and end of sessions (2.97 out of 10), anxiety levels were reduced by 1.65. There is also a decrease of 0.75 in average anxiety scores between reported past week anxiety levels (5.37 out of 10) and anxiety at the start of the session (4.62 out of 10). Table 15.3 shows that the p values for all three paired score comparisons are $p < 0.0005$, which indicates that the score means are statistically different from each other and results are significant.

The comparisons of anxiety levels at the start and end of each session for all participants is shown in Figure 15.1. The figure shows that anxiety was reduced in the majority of sessions, shown by the majority of sessions leading to the negative numbers in the graph and a 36% reduction average as shown in Table 15.2.

The comparisons of average anxiety levels from the past week and the end of each session for all participants and sessions are shown in Figure 15.2. In contrast to Figure 15.1, Figure 15.2 exhibits longer bars for anxiety reductions of -5 or greater; hence, there are more sessions that show stronger reductions. This matches Table 15.3 above, which reports mean anxiety reductions of 45% after the virtual art therapy sessions when compared to past week values. Furthermore, the bar for no change in anxiety is much shorter in Figure 15.2 than in Figure 15.1, indicating there are about 54 fewer sessions that show no change.

Table 15.4 provides the percentage of virtual art therapy sessions that show a reduction in reported anxiety levels, the same anxiety, and anxiety increase in relation to the total number of sessions (774). It shows that 74% of the sessions exhibit a reduced anxiety rate when comparing anxiety level scores at the end of

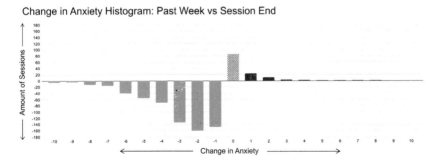

Figure 15.1 CiiAT Anxiety Likert Scale (CALS) Results: Differences in Pre-Post Art Therapy Session Anxiety Levels
Note: Negative values indicate anxiety reduction, whereas positive values indicate an increase in anxiety at the end of the session

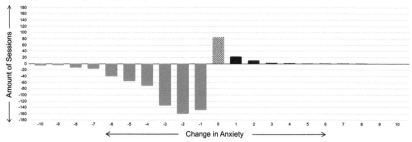

Figure 15.2 CiiAT Anxiety Likert Scale (CALS) Results: Differences in Past Week to Post Art Therapy Session Anxiety Levels
Note: Negative values indicate anxiety reduction, whereas positive values indicate an increase in anxiety at the end of the session

Table 15.4 Percentage of Total Sessions (774) Where Anxiety Was Reduced, Stayed the Same or Increased After Virtual Art Therapy

Comparisons between Client-reported Anxiety Levels	Sessions that show anxiety reduction	Sessions that show same anxiety	Sessions that show anxiety increase
Average reported level of anxiety over past week vs. beginning of art therapy session	49% (376 sessions)	31% (242 sessions)	20% (156 sessions)
Average reported level of anxiety during start of session vs. end of art therapy session	74% (573 sessions)	18% (140 sessions)	8% (61 sessions)
Average reported level of anxiety over past week vs. end of art therapy session	83% (642 sessions)	11% (86 sessions)	6% (46 sessions)

the session versus anxiety scores at the start of the session. Furthermore, 83% of the sessions exhibit reduced anxiety levels between the end of the virtual art therapy sessions and reported anxiety levels over the past week.

Discussion

Student art therapists from the Canadian International Institute of Art Therapy at the Virtual Art Therapy Clinic sought to determine whether attending 60-minute virtual art therapy sessions could reduce subjective reports of anxiety in 87 adult clients over the span of one year. This study used the 10-point CiiAT Anxiety Likert Scale to measure self-reported client anxiety levels over the previous week, at the beginning of the session, and at the end of the online session with an art therapy student. The data collected over a 12-month period

(774 sessions) indicate a reduction in average anxiety scores from past week to session start, past week to session end, and session start to session end. The student therapists reported that they did not encounter significant problems administering art therapy online.

This research contributes to the growing body of literature on art therapy through videoconferencing (Jones et al., 2018; Levy et al., 2018; Malchiodi, 2018; Shaw, 2020). This pilot study can provide insight into whether individual virtual art therapy sessions can reduce anxiety with adult clients and expand upon this art therapy research for adults across the globe.

The results of this study suggest that a single, 60-minute session of virtual art therapy can significantly (p < 0.0005 for all three t-tests) reduce adult clients' reported levels of anxiety pre-and post-session. The data indicates an important shift in average anxiety scores before and after a 60-minute virtual art therapy session with an art therapist student. The answers to CALS questions at session start and session end, which assessed subjective reports of anxiety (with 0 being no anxiety and 10 being the highest), showed a 36% reduction from a 4.62 mean score to a 2.97 mean score. When looking at the past week score, it was lowered even further by 45% from 5.37 to 2.97 at session end. Furthermore, there was a smaller reduction of 14% between the mean past week score 5.37 and the beginning of the session 4.62.

The collective data show that 74% of the sessions exhibit a reduced anxiety rate when comparing the average anxiety levels at the end of the session to the average anxiety levels at the beginning of sessions. Furthermore, 83% of the sessions exhibit a reduced anxiety rate when comparing the average anxiety score over the last week to the average anxiety score at the end of the session. About half the sessions (49%) indicate a reduction in anxiety at the beginning of the session when compared to the past week's score. This shows that there is a therapeutic effect simply by seeking out help, but the effect is not as strong as undergoing art therapy, which can be seen by the much larger and more frequent anxiety reduction by session end.

The anxiety levels at the beginning of the sessions had a greater variance than reported anxiety over the past week or at the end of the session. This may be because clients reporting their anxiety levels at the beginning of the session may have been influenced by factors immediately preceding the session, such as a family crisis at home or work stress, rather than a retrospective report of longer-term anxiety levels over the week.

The act of asking the three questions held a therapeutic value for some clients because it allowed them to realize their own progress. It was also beneficial for student therapists, according to in-person communications. It became an immediate gauge or marker of the client's experience of anxiety at that moment, a gauge that the student therapist might not have otherwise ascertained. Utilizing the CALS had the potential to invite the therapist to reflect on the effectiveness of the session, through conversation with the client directly, private reflection and response art, and between student therapist and clinical supervisor after the session.

Eight percent of the art therapy sessions increased clients' anxiety levels when comparing anxiety scores at session end with those at session start. This did not surprise researchers. As most art therapists understand from clinical experience, art making can escalate anxiety for any number of reasons. In this study, for example, had the student therapist initiated an art activity that contributed to the client's increased anxiety? Did the client work with specific art materials that evoked stressful or traumatic memories? Was there a brief mismatch in the therapeutic alliance—an uncomfortable interaction or a missed opportunity to provide an emotionally corrective experience? Were there technical problems or internet connection issues that caused frustration? While data was not collected on the possible reasons contributing to increased anxiety from beginning to the end of the session, they became learning opportunities for the students in this practicum setting.

In contrast, this study shows a reduction in anxiety in 74% of the sessions when comparing the anxiety score at the beginning of the session with the score at the end. Although there are many factors at play during therapy, this reduction may highlight the positive effects of art therapy as clients find release through creative expression regarding the emotions and stressors that contribute to anxiety.

Furthermore, when comparing the difference in anxiety scores between the past week and the beginning of the session, in about half the sessions (49%) clients felt less anxious at the beginning of the session. This indicates that clients may feel better simply knowing they have a scheduled therapy session. It may indicate the power of the therapeutic alliance; when clients feel connected to their therapists, they have a sense of anticipation that may reduce their anxiety. People feel hopeful when they are about to spend an hour with someone who supports them. The anticipation itself may have a calming effect.

In line with prior teletherapy studies, researchers in this CiiAT study identified the following potential benefits of delivering art therapy online:

- Reducing the stress of commuting to sessions for clients who experience high anxiety
- Easy access for clients with mobility challenges and disabilities
- Increased attendance
- The ability to work with clients internationally
- Freedom to share regarding sexual issues, identity, suicidal thoughts or ideation, infidelity, political opinions, protests, which may be stigmatized in the client's culture
- The safety of a screen is a barrier between the therapist and the client
- Use of art materials that clients are comfortable within their homes.

Limitations

The number of participants in this study (87) is small and therefore results cannot be generalized. Although about 1,400 sessions were completed within the 12-month study, sessions with incomplete data and sessions with clients under the age of 18 and couples were excluded, leaving 774 sessions. Jane was not equipped for automated data collection. Students were encouraged to ask clients the three questions without bias, pressure, or a desired outcome, but it was not possible to eliminate bias. Also, the study only reports the first 12 months of using CALS, which is not a standardized questionnaire. The results cannot be readily compared with results from other anxiety studies.

Furthermore, art therapy via videoconferencing may not work for all clients due to digital fatigue and stress from being on a computer for a long time (Malchiodi, 2018; Riedl et al., 2012). Additionally, virtual art therapy is not accessible to all individuals, as some people do not own computers or smartphones, are uncomfortable with technology, or may not have the internet bandwidth to sustain a videoconferencing call (Jones et al., 2018; Malchiodi, 2018; Usiskin & Lloyd, 2020; Walls, 2018). This "digital divide" (van Dijk, 2006) can deter people from lower-income levels or older adults from engaging in virtual art therapy (Malchiodi, 2018). Further studies should address these technological inequities to access virtual art therapy.

Finally, participants were not qualitatively asked why they experienced a reduction of anxiety at the beginning or after virtual art therapy sessions. Therefore, the underlying causes of this reduction of self-reported anxiety levels is unknown. Anxiety could be reduced due to conversations with the student art therapist, art making, sitting, or sharing emotions in a safe space (among other art therapy-related phenomena). Therefore, qualitative studies and arts-based studies that look at the nature of experiences of COVID-19 stress and virtual art therapy are needed.

The research presented here provides a preliminary snapshot and should be expanded upon with more adult clients and greater session numbers. Therefore, the CiiAT Virtual Art Therapy Clinic will continue with this research and take into account some of the gaps and limitations that were observed during the course of this pilot study.

Conclusion

With the global pandemic increasing fear of illness and significantly changing how people live since March 2020, the mental health of the world has been impacted (World Health Organization, 2020b; Statistics Canada, 2020). A need for accessible and safe mental health support that addresses the impacts of COVID-19 on mental health, such as anxiety, has been identified (World Health Organization, 2020b; Statistics Canada, 2020).

The purpose of this quasi-experimental pilot study was to examine whether student-led virtual art therapy conducted with videoconferencing technology could alleviate anxiety in adult clients. The anxiety levels of clients who registered with the Virtual Art Therapy Clinic, administered by 15 Canadian International Institute of Art Therapy masters-level students, were assessed pre- and post-art therapy sessions for 12 months with a 3-question, 10-point Likert scale, the CiiAT Anxiety Likert Scale. The research study found a 36% reduction of average self-reported anxiety levels at the beginning (4.62 out of 10) and after (2.97 out of 10) the art therapy sessions, when clients were asked to share their current feeling of anxiety on a scale from one to ten. Furthermore, the study found a reduction of 45% when comparing the reported anxiety over the last week (5.37 out of 10) to the score at the end of the session (2.97 out of 10). Although these results are preliminary and contain a small sample size, they are encouraging and should be expanded upon with a longer-term, large-scale study.

References

Abbing, A., Baars, E. W., de Sonneville, L., Ponstein, A. S., & Swaab, H. (2019). The effectiveness of art therapy for anxiety in adult women: A randomized controlled trial. *Frontiers in Psychology, 10*, 1203. https://doi.org/10.3389/fpsyg.2019.01203.

American Psychiatric Association. (2013). *Diagnostic and statistical manual of mental disorders* (5th ed.). https://doi.org/10.1176/appi.books.9780890425596.

Bao, Y., Sun, Y., Meng, S., Shi, J., & Lu, L. (2020). 2019-nCoV epidemic: Address mental health care to empower society. *Lancet, 22*(395), e37–e38. https://www.ncbi.nlm.nih.gov/pmc/articles/PMC7133594/.

Bennett, C. M., Lambie, G. W., Bai, H., & Hundley, G. (2020). Neurofeedback training to address college students' symptoms of anxiety and stress: A quasi-experimental design. *Journal of College Student Psychotherapy.* https://doi.org/10.1080/87568225.2020.1791777.

Berryhill, M., Halli-Tierney, A., Culmer, N., Williams, N., Betancourt, A., King, M., & Ruggles, H. (2019). Videoconferencing psychological therapy and anxiety: A systematic review. *Family Practice, 36*(1), 53–63, https://doi.org/10.1093/fampra/cmy072.

Bringhurst, D. L., Watson, C. W., Miller, S. D., & Duncan, B. L. (2006). The reliability and validity of the Outcome Rating Scale: A replication study of a brief clinical measure. *Journal of Brief Therapy, 5*, 23–30.

Brunier, A. (2016). Investing in treatment for depression and anxiety leads to fourfold return. *World Health Organization.* https://www.who.int/news-room/detail/13-04-2016-investing-in-treatment-for-depression-and-anxiety-leads-to-fourfold-return.

Campbell, A., & Hemsley, S. (2009). Outcome Rating Scale and Session Rating Scale in psychological practice: Clinical utility of ultra-brief measures. *Clinical Psychologist, 13*(1), 1–9. https://doi.org/10.1080/13284200802676391.

Carter, J. D., Crowe, M., Carlyle, D., Frampton, C. M., Jordan, J., McIntosh, V. V. W., O'Toole, V. M., Whitehead, L., & Joyce, P. R. (2011). Patient change processes in psychotherapy: Development of a new scale. *Psychotherapy Research, 22*(1), 115–126. doi:10.1080/10503307.2011.631195.

Chambala, A. (2008). Anxiety and art therapy: Treatment in the public eye. *Art Therapy Journal of the American Art Therapy Association, 25*(4) 187–189.

Collie, K., & Čubranić, D. (1999). An art therapy solution to a telehealth problem. *Art Therapy 16*(4), 186–193.

Curry, N., & Kasser, T. (2005). Can coloring mandalas reduce anxiety? *Art Therapy, 22*(2), 81–85.

Czamanski-Cohen, J., & Weihs, K. (2016). The bodymind model: A platform for studying the mechanisms of change induced by art therapy. *The Arts in Psychotherapy, 51*, 63–71. https://www.ncbi.nlm.nih.gov/pmc/articles/PMC5074079/.

Davey, H. M., Barratt, A. L., Butow, P. N., & Deeks, J., J. (2007). A one-item question with a Likert or Visual Analog Scale adequately measured current anxiety. *Journal of Clinical Epidemiology, 60*(4), 356–360. https://pubmed.ncbi.nlm.nih.gov/17346609/.

Dew, A., Smith, L., Collings, S., & Isabella, D. S. (2018). Complexity embodied: Using body mapping to understand complex support needs. *Forum: Qualitative Social Research, 19*(2), 1–25.

Government of Canada (2020, November 26). Coronavirus disease (COVID-19): Outbreak update. *Government of Canada.* https://www.canada.ca/en/public-health/services/diseases/2019-novel-coronavirus-infection.html.

Harris, A. D., McGregor, J. C., Perencevich, Furuno, E. N., Zhu, J., Peterson, D. E., & Finkelstein, J. (2006). The use and interpretation of quasi-experimental studies in medical informatics. *Journal of the American Medical Informatics Association, 13*(1). 16–23. https://doi.org/10.1197/jamia.M1749.

Hass-Cohen, N., & Findlay, C. J. (2015). *Art therapy and the neuroscience of relationships, creativity, and resiliency.* Norton & Company.

Howlett, M. (2021). Looking at the 'field' through a Zoom lens: Methodological reflections on conducting online research during a global pandemic. *Qualitative Research.* https://doi.org/10.1177/1468794120985691.

Jane Software Inc. (2020a). Online Appointments is Live. https://jane.app/guide/telehealth/online-appointments-is-live.

Jane Software Inc. (2020b). Is Jane PIPEDA Compliant?https://jane.app/guide/privacy-and-security/is-jane-pipeda-compliant.

Jones, G. (2017, April 17). Providing art therapy in palliative care using telehealth technology. *British Association of Art Therapists.* https://www.baat.org/About-BAAT/Blog/121/Providing-Art-Therapy-in-Palliative-Care-using-Telehealth-Technology.

Jones, G., Rahman, R., & Robson, M. (2018). Group art therapy and telemedicine. In C. Malchiodi (Ed.), *The handbook of art therapy and digital technology* (pp. 303–316). Jessica Kingsley Publishers.

Joint Task Force for the Development of Telepsychology Guidelines for Psychologists. (2013). Guidelines for the practice of telepsychology . *American Psychological Association, 68*(9), 791–800. https://doi.org/10.1037/a0035001.

Kaimal, G., Ray, K., & Muniz, J. (2016). Reduction of cortisol levels and participants' responses following art-making. *Art Therapy: Journal of the American Art Therapy Association, 33*(2), 74–80.

Kaimal, G., Mensinger, J. L., Drass, J. M., & Dieterich-Hartwell, R. M. (2017) Art therapist-facilitated open studio versus coloring: Differences in outcomes of affect, stress, creative agency, and self-efficacy. *Canadian Art Therapy Association Journal, 30*(2), 56–68. https://doi.org/10.1080/08322473.2017.1375827.

Kapitan, L. (2018). *Introduction to art therapy research.* Taylor & Francis.

Kendall-Tackett, K. (2020). A social history of the coronavirus. *Psychological Trauma: Theory, Research, Practice, and Policy, 12*(S1), S1–S2. http://dx.doi.org/10.1037/tra0000955.

Kirkey, S. (2018, October 29). Nearly half of Canadians report struggling with anxiety, but are we really coming undone? *The National Post.* https://nationalpost.com/hea lth/its-not-just-you-nearly-half-of-canadians-struggling-with-anxiety-but-are-we-rea lly-coming-undon.

Laurer, M., & van der Vennet, R. (2015). Effect of art production on negative mood and anxiety for adults in treatment for substance abuse. *Art Therapy, 32*(4), 173–183.

Levy, C., Spooner, H., Lee, J., Sonke, J., Myers, K., & Snow, E. (2018). Telehealth-based creative arts therapy: Transforming mental health and rehabilitation care for rural veterans. *The Arts in Psychotherapy, 57.* https://doi.org/10.1016/j.aip.2017.08.010.

Malchiodi, C. (2007). *The art therapy sourcebook.* McGraw-Hill.

Malchiodi, C. (2017). Creative arts therapies and arts-based research. In P. Leavy (Ed.), *Handbook of arts-based research* (pp. 68–87). Guilford Press.

Malchiodi, C. (2018). Appendix 1: General ethical potential principals for cyber art therapists. In C. Malchiodi (Ed.), *The handbook of art therapy and digital technology* (pp. 391–393). Jessica Kingsley Publishers.

Mental Health Research Canada. (2020, December). Mental Health During COVID-19 Outbreak: Poll #4 of 13 in a Series (Mid-December Data Collection). https://www.mhrc.ca/national-data-on-covid.

Miller, G., & McDonald, A. (2020). Online art therapy during the COVID-19 pandemic, *International Journal of Art Therapy, 25*(4), 159–160. https://10.1080/17454832.2020.1846383.

National Institute of Mental Health. (2018, July). Anxiety Disorders. https://www.nimh.nih.gov/health/topics/anxiety-disorders/index.shtml.

Potash, J. S., Kalmanowitz, D., Fund, I., Anand, S. A., & Miller, G. M. (2020). Art therapy in pandemics: Lessons for COVID-19. *Art Therapy, 37*(2), 105–107.

Proulx Global Education and Community Foundation. (2021). Virtual Art Therapy Clinic. https://arttherapy.network/.

Rajkumar, R. P. (2020). COVID-19 and mental health: A review of the existing literature. *Asian Journal of Psychiatry, 52.* https://doi.org/10.1016/j.ajp.2020.102066.

Riedl, R., Kindermann, H., Auinger, A., & Javor, A. (2012). Technostress from a neurobiological perspective. *Business and Information Systems Engineering 4*(2), 61–69.

Sandmire, D. A., Gorham, S. R., Rankin, N. E., & Grimm, D. R. (2012). The influence of art making on anxiety: A pilot study. *Art Therapy, 29*(2), 68–73. httsp://doi.org/10.1080/07421656.2012.683748.

Shaw, L. (2020). 'Don't look!' An online art therapy group for adolescents with Anorexia Nervosa. *International Journal of Art Therapy, 25*(4), 211–217. https://doi.org/10.1080/17454832.2020.1845757.

Shella, T. A. (2018). Art therapy improves mood, and reduces pain and anxiety when offered at bedside during acute hospital treatment. *The Arts in Psychotherapy, 57,* 59–64. https://doi.org/10.1016/j.aip.2017.10.003.

Sherrington, C. S. (1906). *Integrative actions of the nervous system.* Yale University Press: New Haven.

Spitzer R. L., Kroenke K., Williams J. B. W., Löwe B. (2006). A brief measure for assessing generalized anxiety disorder the GAD-7. *Archives of Internal Medicine, 166,* 1092–1097.

Statistics Canada (2020, May 27) Canadians' Mental Health During the COVID-19 Pandemic (Stats Can Publication No. 11–001-X). Government of Canada, Statistics Canada. https://www150.statcan.gc.ca/n1/daily-quotidien/200527/dq200527b-eng.pdf.

Usiskin, M., & Lloyd, B. (2020) Lifeline, frontline, online: Adapting art therapy for social engagement across borders. *International Journal of Art Therapy*, *25*(4), 183–191. https://doi.org/10.1080/17454832.2020.1845219.

van der Kolk, B. (2014). *The Body keeps the score: Brain, mind, and body in the healing of trauma.* Penguin.

van Dijk, J. A. G. M. (2006). Digital divide research, achievements and shortcomings. *Poetics*, *34*(4–5), 221–235. https://doi.org/10.1016/j.poetic.2006.05.004.

Visnola, D., Sprūdža, D., Ārija Baķe, M., & Piķe, A. (2010). Effects of art therapy on stress and anxiety of employees. *Proceedings of the Latvian Academy of Sciences. Section B. Natural, Exact, and Applied Sciences*, *64*(1–2), 85–91. https://doi.org/10.2478/v10046-010-0020-y.

Walls, J. (2018). A telehealth primer for art therapy. In C. Malchiodi (Ed.), *The handbook of art therapy and digital technology* (pp. 159–174). Jessica Kingsley Publishers.

Wang, C., Pan, R., Wan, X., Tan, Y., Xu, L., Ho, C. S., & Ho, R. C. (2020). Immediate psychological responses and associated factors during the initial stage of the 2019 coronavirus disease (COVID-19) epidemic among the general population in China. *International Journal of Environmental Research and Public Health*, *17*(5) (2020). E1729. https://www.mdpi.com/1660-4601/17/5/1729/htm.

World Health Organization (2020a). Timeline: WHO's COVID-19 response. *World Health Organization*. https://www.who.int/emergencies/diseases/novel-coronavirus-2019/interactive-timeline.

World Health Organization (2020b, May 13). Policy Brief: Covid-19 and the need for action on mental health. *World Health Organization*. https://www.un.org/sites/un2.un.org/files/un_policy_brief-covid_and_mental_health_final.pdf.

Xiao, H., Zhang, Y., Kong, D., Li, S., & Yang, N. (2020). The effects of social support on sleep quality of medical staff treating patients with coronavirus disease 2019 (COVID-19) in January and February 2020 in China. *Medical Science Monitor: International Medical Journal of Experimental and Clinical Research*, *26*, e923549.

Section 4

Virtual Vistas

16 Art Therapy with Virtual Reality

Christel Bodenbender

WITH EXCERPTS FROM INTERVIEWS WITH I. HACMUN AND G. KAIMAL CONDUCTED
BY THE CANADIAN INTERNATIONAL INSTITUTE OF ART THERAPY IN NOVEMBER 2020

Introduction

I was often the odd one in the art therapy class—the one who preferred art making in a digital environment over the traditional paint-on-canvas. Both can be fun, but digital art gave me the freedom to let go of my worries that the next stroke could ruin everything I had created, because with the help of the *undo* function, I could always go back to the previous state. Hence, I kept my gaze on technological developments and their art-making potentials.

Lifting us up from a two-dimensional canvas into a three-dimensional world, Virtual Reality (VR) technology has given us a new tool to create art in a digital environment, as VR enables human interactions in a computer-generated simulation (Kaimal et al., 2019, p. 16). The first time I put on a VR headset was at a science-fiction convention in the 1990s. I was mesmerized by the way I could interact with the digital environment through the haptic glove and alter my view through head movements; yet, at the same time, I was disappointed by the clunky graphics and limited range of motion. The experience left a lasting impression. I wanted to experience more and better versions of it, and followed advances in VR technology through the news.

In 2019, I bought an Oculus Quest VR head-mounted display and controllers. I chose this device because the Oculus Quest is a self-contained unit that does not involve any cables to an external computer, which I considered a hindrance to a client's movements. I also purchased the software Google Tilt Brush and began to draw in an immersive, virtual, three-dimensional environment that was worlds beyond the 1990s with regard to interactive immediacy while maintaining visual quality. Maybe *draw* is not the right word—I find a term like *sculpt* might be a better fit since most of the artwork stretches in three dimensions, more akin to a sculpture than a flat drawing on a piece of paper. Similarly, Hacmun et al. (2018, VR Creative Environment) argue that drawing in VR combines forms of painting (i.e. line, shape, and colour) with the three-dimensional element of sculpting as well as new digital possibilities, such as making strokes that glow and dynamically vibrate like lightning.

DOI: 10.4324/9781003149538-20

I tried out the Oculus Quest and Tilt Brush with some friends and relatives, watching their art-making process as I streamed their point of view onto a tablet. The digital natives, in particular, told me how much they liked the experience. It was fun and they enjoyed the ability to move around in the art making space, and around and even through their artwork. I could hear the pride in their voices, which, for me, hinted at the emotional engagement and therapeutic opportunity of VR art making.

My consecutive attempt to find clients by advertising myself as a VR Art Therapist, however, were met with limited success. Maybe clients were not yet ready for VR art therapy—at least not the people I reached with my posters in the town where I lived. My mistake might also have been that I had advertised my vision as VR Art Therapy specifically, instead of Art Therapy *with* VR. As Hacmun pointed out in her interview with the Canadian International Institute of Art Therapy (CiiAT) in 2020,

> I think it is important for me to say this is not VR art therapy; this is art therapy with another medium called VR. A client can use the VR and then compliment it with another medium. In the end, it is what the client needs that is being addressed.

Many adults, however, seldom do art. In her interview with CiiAT in 2020, Kaimal spoke about clients from Western society: "I'll meet someone in a session, and they'll say to me, 'The last time I held a pencil or a crayon was in elementary school,' and these are people in their sixties or seventies." My assumption that the general population would readily embrace art making along with an unfamiliar technology may have been a few hurdles too many for my vision to work despite growing evidence that VR offers a novel tool to the field of art therapy that should not be as easily dismissed. Hacmun said,

> This space in ... VR, where you can create—it's the perfect potential space. It's playful. It's dreamy, even for people who are not so playful.... . When I imagine Winnicott's *potential space* (i.e., a place of creative playing), this is how I imagine it.

With VR adoption gaining steam with consumers, Liu & Chang (2018) and Kaimal et al. (2019), for instance, have provided experimental studies that researched virtual reality technology in art therapy that will be addressed in this chapter.

I do not advocate that every art therapist needs to be passionate about each art-making tool, but the art therapy field as a whole has to consider how to best reach and engage each single client, which may include art making through VR systems as discussed in this chapter. As Hacmun stressed, "The debate of whether to use it or not [is] not just to stay relevant; it's to serve our clients better because they are changing."

Virtual Reality Technology as an Art Making Tool

Creative expression has been part of human history since ivory carvings and early cave paintings, expressing symbolic thought (D'Arcy, 2017) and what seems like a reflection of previous lived experiences and beliefs. Over the course of history, art making has changed and been expanded with the development of new technologies, such as better tools, extraction of more colours, and the development of paper and printmaking. With technological progress, novel digital, art-making media have emerged that are explored by art therapists to benefit clients, such as using VR devices.

Virtual reality refers to an immersion in a virtual world through a head gear that includes a head-mounted display (sight) and speakers (sound) as well as the use of hand-held, wireless controllers to interact with objects in the virtual world (see Figure 16.1).

With sight and hearing immersed in the virtual world, the person wearing the headset appears to move and act in the physical world, but generally remains conscious of being in a virtual world since touch is limited to the plastic of the controllers, smell remains in the real world, and graphics still lack the depth of the natural world. It is, thus, an imaginary experience and yet more sophisticated and realistic than content presented on our phone and computer screens. Liu and Chang have identified high-level immersion as the primary attraction for the participants in their study on art therapy with VR (2018, p. 49). Hacmun noted that by

> using a VR headset, you know you are in virtual reality but you cannot escape the new reality within the headset. It becomes something you experience that feels real. Even for fun, you can do online virtual reality roller coasters and you can see a physical immersive response in people.

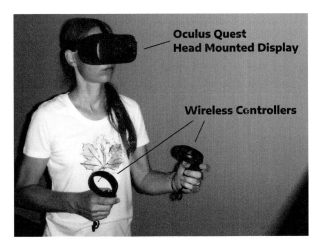

Figure 16.1 Wearing the Oculus Quest Head Gear and Controllers

This is how you check for immersivity—you can see the physical reaction to the virtual reality they are seeing.

The virtual environment is assembled by a combination of software and hardware that provide the illusion of the three-dimensional world and the tools to interact with and modify this world. Liu and Chang (2018) and Kaimal et al. (2019) have studied the use of Google's Tilt Brush software as an artistic medium that allows study participants to express loss and sadness, manage emotions, and release pressure. I have also explored Tilt Brush and have found the art-making capabilities extensive with the many tools that are provided. Developed in 2016, Tilt Brush's three-dimensional virtual drawing environment consists of an adaptable surrounding, where the user can choose between different settings, an art material palette that is accessed through the controller in the left hand, and the brush, which is managed through the controller in the right hand (see Figure 16.2).

The user can choose between a wide selection of digital brushes, which range from paint-like strokes to a streak of sparkling stars, a colour selection, and tools, such as importing images and a teleporter to quickly move through the virtual environment. Furthermore, the digital space and the created objects are scalable, which means the user can shrink and expand artwork with the controllers. Created works can be saved to the device and revisited in a later session. It is a private space, controlled by the client within the parameters of the software. Even when clients may feel out of control in their lives, they have full control here. At the same time, the software allows the therapist to follow and revisit the art-making steps through repeated viewing, which benefits the therapy (Liu & Chang, 2018, p. 49), as discussed in the following section.

Art Therapy and Virtual Reality

Art therapy attempts to present "emotional conflicts and personality development in subconscious minds through artistic expression … [by focusing] on an inward view and emotional release" (Liu & Chang, 2018, p. 48). Art therapists traditionally rely on the expressive modalities that have a proven track record for their therapeutic value. However, the more digital technologies become part of our

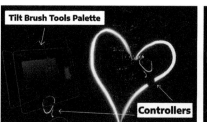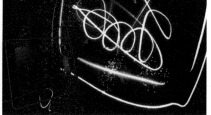

Figure 16.2 VR Point-of-View: 2 Screenshots of Tilt Brush Drawing Environment

lives, the more their creative potential becomes relevant to clients as part of their lived experiences. Regarding the adoption of VR in art therapy, Hacmun said, "There is a long-lasting debate concerning digital mediums—can they be considered for art? Do they possess artistic qualities for art therapy although they lack sensation and form?"[1]

For instance, Kaimal et al.'s study indicates "that creative expression in VR can help reduce inhibitions, activate full-body movements, and enhance mood and creative play exploration … [as it] engaged kinesthetic, visual, and aural senses in the art-making process" (2019, pp. 17–18). The play and exploration was reported as "intuitive" with "endless possibilities" taking place in "a calm space" (p. 18). Most study participants enjoyed leaving behind the constraints of the physical world, such as by moving through objects in the virtual world. Overall, participants reported a positive experience and even joy and euphoria. Furthermore, Kaimal et al. observed that when traditional art materials were used following the VR experience, the range of expression was altered as "participants used the artwork created in VR as a source of inspiration" (p. 21). Kaimal added in the interview,

> Maybe it's a novelty aspect, but when we have people come into VR, they are so energized. They are shaken up, but in a good way, usually. We had one person who felt nauseous and uncomfortable, but most people come out rejuvenated and revitalized.

As an added benefit, Kaimal et al. identified VR as a potential tool "to facilitate self-expression among patients unable to engage in activities requiring fine motor control and to help patients in immune-compromised environments as well as those uncomfortable with the excessive sensory stimulation of art media" (2019, p. 21). Furthermore, Hacmun identified a lower threshold for artistic skill in VR in general. She stated,

> In VR we have qualities like 3-D painting. It is different from painting. You don't need the rules of perspective. You don't need to do the lines in a way that looks like reality in 2D. One of the tasks we sometimes give, just for fun, is to draw a cube. They struggle with it because they do it like they are trying to draw on paper but soon learn how to use the 3-D space and find it is very easy. It is very intuitive. You don't have to think or see what it looks like—you just draw and move around. There is this quality of very intuitive drawing. When we think about people [who] are very afraid of drawing, clients that are focused on results, this is a space where you can't go wrong.

One feature of digital art is the flexibility to go back to a previous version of the artwork through the *undo* function, reinstating a previously saved state, or selecting and erasing a particular stroke or element. Personally, this is one of the primary features that attracted me to digital art making. I find it liberating to be able to go back to a previous state, which makes exploration free of regretting a stroke and free of the fear of failure. In life, I cannot go back in time and have a better past, as much as I may dream about it. In digital art, however, I can return the artwork to a previous state and, with the knowledge of the steps that did not work or did not lead to satisfying results, I can do things differently, proving to myself that I have the power to do things right. Kaimal explained,

> If you think about someone who feels stuck or trapped, when you put them through the VR experience, which challenges everything they know to be true, [it] allows them to explore without fear of failure. We don't allow ourselves to fail enough, and therefore we become afraid. We become afraid to try things. Digital tools take away that fear of failure because you can undo everything.

VR, thus, provides a stage to experiment freely. Hacmun noted that whereas

> classic materials are rigid or flexible, VR can be both. Creation with VR can be very expressive involving body movements or it can be controlled. When we consider the Expressive Therapies Continuum, VR offers us an opportunity of fluidity, to work flexibly, and move freely along the scales while best suiting the client's needs.

The immediate scalability of the created artwork or an art element can have profound therapeutic effects as you can stretch and shrink objects with a few clicks in Tilt Brush. Hacmun illustrated this point:

> Think about a monster drawn on paper as done in many classical artistic interventions. Here, in VR, you can make it larger and you can feel it because you are inside the virtual environment with it. You can then make it tiny and feel it being tiny. You have a whole different experience with the artwork; it is embodied and more three-dimensional.

Because of the depth of the VR canvas, creative expression with Tilt Brush allows us to combine a wide range of body movements with the creation process. As previously mentioned, art making in VR feels more like sculpting than drawing. Although you can also choose to paint a surface in the VR world, art objects typically take shape in a three-dimensional space rather than on the surface of a two-dimensional canvas. I watched some of the people who tried out my VR system move their entire body up and down, swaying from side to side as they drew. Their arms went all the way up, as far as they could stretch, and back down to the floor. They were able to walk around—and even through—their creation, gaining new perspectives from every angle.

Hacmun said about VR and the aspect of movement:

> It's not like how you are used to drawing and creating. Your movements are larger and you can move around 360 degrees.... . In a way, you are

not standing next to a wall or table and limited to a defined size of canvas. VR facilitates big movements and embodied expressions. There is something more holistic in this form of creation. It combines several creative forms, several expressions.

Liu and Chang (2018) regard this engagement of the body in VR as akin to dance movement therapy, which has an "influence on the integrity of self-development and social personality" (p. 49). To enhance the therapeutic process, the therapist can set up the VR system to stream the client's point of view to an external two-dimensional screen, such as a tablet. This allows him or her to follow the art-making process live and provide suggestions (Kaimal et al., 2019, p. 17). Alternatively, the therapist can also choose a third-person perspective (Hacmun et al., 2018, VR Creative Environment). Tilt Brush records the art-making steps and allows every brushstroke to be reviewed, which provides new possibilities for reflection.

Hacmun noted that allowing the therapists to view the VR artwork from the client's point of view

> was excellent for the therapists. In our research, we found it filled a lot of gaps in things that are lacking in the VR therapeutic setting, like the lack of eye contact and visible facial expressions between therapist and client. The therapist felt much closer to the client's experience. As for transference and countertransference, everything was similar. The therapist was not dissolved inside the other's experience. As trained therapists, they were used to this and could get closer without getting too close. It's a wonderful way to be more inside the client's world.

Thus, with the therapist seeing the point of view of the client, this brings a different level of immediacy to the therapist experiencing the art-making process than simply sitting at a table next to a client and watching them from the side.

Regarding whom to invite to art therapy with VR, Hacmun recommended clients from the "general normative population." Particularly, offering art making with VR to adolescents may serve as a gateway because this population can be resistant to traditional art therapy. She further stressed the suitability of VR for digital natives, youth at risk, people who struggle with their imagination, or people who have problems with perspective and mentalization. Putting them into the VR environment provides an immediate level of engagement since clients are immersed in the environment and can build something in an instant. Hacmun noted that wearing the headset can be very helpful for people with low self-esteem or anxieties because it creates the illusion that they are in their own world. She added, however, that in the findings, there was a debate among art therapists regarding the VR potential for people on the autistic spectrum due to the powerful immersive quality of the VR medium. For instance, De Luca et al. (2021) explored a combined treatment method of Cognitive Behavioural Therapy (CBT) and VR in children on the autistic spectrum and found an improvement in spatial cognition skills and attention processes over only using CBT. In contrast, Mesa-Gresa et al.'s (2018) literature review revealed only moderate evidence that VR-based treatments are effective for Autism Spectrum Disorder.

Limitations

One hurdle for using VR in art therapy is that the therapist needs to be proficient enough in the medium in order to provide an introduction and help clients with tool-related questions. In addition, the space for the art therapy session needs to be large enough for clients to move around unobstructed. If space is limited, clients could, instead, sit on a chair and only move their arms. The same applies to clients with mobility restrictions. Both of these cases, however, would benefit from the teleporter function in a VR program, such as Tilt Brush. With this Tilt Brush tool, they can proceed through the virtual space and around objects without having to physically move in the real world, thus giving them a wide range of motion. Furthermore, the controller allows them to grab objects, pull them closer or push them away, and quickly change their size.

Hacmun also warns us about the downsides of the extensive scalability. She said,

> Scalability gives us a movement in perspective as we can see things from different angles—not just different angles, but different sizes. We can see what things are made of and we can enlarge them and enter them. This can also be tricky. It can be really overstimulating; the pace of perspective change is in the nature of the medium itself. As therapists, we have to be aware of the inherent shifts in perspective to be suitable to the client's pace.

She added that

> we have to be aware of the potential of overstimulating the client. We have to know that maybe some clients will need to be sitting in a chair and to go more slowly, or we ... have to pin the canvas so it cannot move. As therapists, it is important to know the medium; it might be very fascinating, but we also have to know how to master the medium and make the experience safe and relaxed.

In this context, we can remind clients that, however real the VR experience appears, they can remove the gear to bring their awareness back to the physical world, offering a grounding resource. Hacmun used the example of a rollercoaster ride: unlike being on a real rollercoaster, you can always remove yourself from the experience in VR by just taking off the head mounted display.

Because of the unfamiliar nature of the technology for most clients, she advised against starting a therapeutic relationship with VR. For Hacmun,

> We found the timing of the presentation of VR into the therapy is after there is an alliance. Maybe in the future, when there is much more experience and we have different protocols, then it will be easier. I would not run into the first session with VR.

This might explain why my attempt at offering VR art therapy did not find enough interest in the general population, because I did not promise a therapeutic alliance first before introducing VR to the sessions. My poster and fliers did not provide that depth of information regarding the nature of the session. Since marketing encourages brevity, buzz words, and graphics, I had planned to talk about the processes involved in a VR art therapy session when potential clients contacted me.

Kaimal et al. (2019) reported that study participants needed time to adjust to the virtual environment, considering that they were unable to see their own bodies. Additionally, there was a similar adjustment when taking the gear off and returning to reality. Using the gear and software involved a learning curve, such as switching between drawing tools, using the eraser, or grabbing objects in the VR space with the controller. This familiarization was mitigated with the help of the therapist and "mirrored the developmental aspects of learning a new art medium" (p. 20).

In the virtual space, study participants only see the controllers, represented by the drawing tool and palette, but not their physical bodies. A few study participants reported this as disorienting (Kaimal et al., 2019, p. 19). On the other hand, the withdrawal of the senses from the real world can serve to block out distractions; clients can forget that they are in a therapy room (Liu & Chang, 2018, p. 49). There is "a sense of privacy and disentanglement from the external world" (Hacmun et al., 2018, The Potential Virtual Space) that can benefit therapy.

Presently, the therapist cannot enter the same virtual space; rather, they can only watch it on a two-dimensional screen. This prevents the potential for co-creation and impacts the nature of the therapeutic interaction (Kaimal et al., 2019, p. 22), with the client only hearing—but not seeing—the therapist. Hacmun explained,

> The basic role of the therapist remains the same, but there are some technical aspects that affect the therapeutic setting. When you put the headset on, you can't see what is happening under there. There is no eye contact or ability to see facial expressions. In the research, some therapists said they didn't need eye contact. For example, when a client sits and does artwork, there isn't any eye contact... . There is no eye contact over the phone [and yet] the core aspects of therapy do not change.

We may have to be cautious when using VR with clients who suffer from hallucinations and delusions because of the realistic qualities of the virtual environment (Kaimal et al., 2019, p. 21). This mirrors studies on using fluid art media, such as watercolour, for clients with psychosis. Hacmun commented,

> I think my assumption is to be more cautious with populations that have problems with reality, who are more confused about reality. Combine it with the immersive quality of the medium and there are still a lot of unknowns that require caution... . Other therapeutic approaches have been treating schizophrenia with VR and have [had] a lot of success.

The studies discussed in this chapter, however, have not included a wide range of participants with different cognitive and physical conditions and abilities. More studies are needed to fill these gaps.

Some study participants were unhappy with "the lack of tangible physical engagement" (Kaimal et al., 2019, p. 19), which included the disappointment over the absence of a physical object that they could take home at the end of therapy sessions. If they choose to take with them an image of the artwork, it misses the three-dimensional qualities that they encountered during the art-making process. Although a three-dimensional print of the artwork may solve this problem, it does not capture all the features of the brush strokes, such as the glow or sparkle effects, and can differ significantly in scale. The lack of a physical object, however, makes it easier for the therapist to keep the artwork between sessions because it can be easily stored on the VR device.

Currently, the tactile experience is limited to feeling the plastic of the controllers, similar to holding a can to spray paint (Hacmun et al., 2018, paragraph 7). The Oculus Quest controllers provide haptic feedback—i.e. a sense of touch—for some of the games through rapid vibration, such as when a player is being hit by an object. This type of feedback in VR increases the sense of presence for the user (Blenkinsopp, n.d., paragraph 17). Regarding art making in Tilt Brush, Hacmun said,

> Currently, there is no haptic feedback—not even vibrations like in gaming... . [Yet], the participants felt the materials to be tangible. Around 90% of them were initially not so keen on the lack of physical touch in the VR medium but, surprisingly, they all said it felt tangible. It felt real. There is something synesthesia-like—a transformation from when you get the visual stimuli and it gets transferred to another sense. There is something happening inside. Because of the quality and immersivity, there is a synesthesia-like feeling, creating a sense of haptic feedback.

The artwork produced in a VR environment may not be a tactile element of the real world, but it still exists as an image, just like a drawn pipe is not a pipe and yet we recognize it as a pipe in our minds. Ultimately, our perception of the world is based on sensory information fed to our brains and supplemented by our thoughts and dreams about it. A virtual reality experience is as valid an experience as getting out of bed in the morning. For art therapy to work, it comes down to what the experience does for the client's healing journey.

Visions of the Future

This chapter focuses on VR, but there are similar efforts in developing Augmented Reality (AR), which also involves a head-mounted display, such as the Microsoft Hololens, and could be utilized in art therapy with programs like Tilt Brush. As Hacmun explained,

> AR, compared to VR, is different by the ratio of how much reality is inside. Augmented reality uses reality as the foundation plus something virtual on top, thereby augmenting reality. Virtual reality is totally a simulation … it can be fantasy-like or real-like but it is not real. Currently, virtual reality is more developed and advanced technically. There are a lot more options with VR. In AR, it is much more difficult to mix the real and unreal.

She added,

> In VR, we have a kind of agreement; when we enter a movie, there is a suspension of disbelief—we enter an agreement to see things that are a little less realistic… . When we see a virtual dragon in VR, we know it is virtual—we are in a fantasy world. But when we see a dragon come out of our wall in AR, it is much more confusing because it is in a place that is real, in our own room. When reality starts being different [from] your everyday life with monsters coming out, for someone less anchored to reality, it can be really frightening because they don't have that agreement: is it real or is it unreal? … I'm not saying AR will not be useful for art therapy, but in general, due to the current technological state, and to be on the safe side of reality monitoring, VR is something we use more now for art therapy.

With further developments in virtual and augmented technologies, a therapist could meet their client in virtual space. They would both share the same space and, although they may be continents apart, they could come together in this space and even do art together. This would be a more direct form of an art therapy tele-treatment than a videoconferencing meeting can offer. Hacmun illustrated during her interview with CiiAT,

> We should have done this meeting in VR. There are virtual spaces to meet, like in a room that gives the feeling like we are there. In VR, you can experience the artwork and meet in a shared space to do it together.

She added that

> you can go and watch a movie with a friend, sitting next to each other in VR with an avatar that represents you. You feel immersed inside of it and you can feel as if you are [truly] watching a movie with a friend.

I hope that art therapy embraces the changes. I think art therapy is a wonderful way to help people. It is a connection to our natural instinct to heal. Even with the tools of the future, there is something fascinating about it. We have a lot of work to do, [and] things are changing all the time. It's also something, in general, for all professions, but art therapy has an opportunity. We see therapies going towards more embodied and experiential. There is the potential to provide better solutions across the board.

Conclusion

As discussed in many chapters of this book, new approaches to art therapy include eco-art therapy, walking studios, and psychogeography, which expand the range of modalities we can use in an art therapy practice. Furthermore, digital media have been explored to engage clients, such as the whiteboard tool within the Zoom videoconference platform, and client sessions have been carried out virtually in addition to in-person. Thus, the field of art therapy does not stand still and with new technologies, novel art-making media must be explored to benefit clients.

With the investigations presented in this chapter, the field of art therapy is striding forward by studying VR as a tool for therapeutic creative expression. Many young people, in particular, are interested in electronic arts (Liu & Chang, 2018, p. 49) as "digital technology is an integrative part of their everyday lives" (Hacmun et al., 2018, Summary). Art therapy with VR, for instance, can be an approach to better reach them on a turf that is more comfortable for them—or to start a session with VR and then intersperse some more tactile experience to access different levels of emotional processing. There are many possible applications for a wide range of populations, including mood enhancement and facilitating self-expression (Kaimal et al, 2019). In the end, it depends on the clients and their needs in each session that determine which art-making tool best serves them that particular time. Art making in VR is here to stay and become part of the art therapy tool box.

Note

1 See the work of Penelope Orr for more information on this discussion.

References

Blenkinsopp, R. (n.d.). *What is haptic feedback?*https://www.ultraleap.com/company/news/blog/what-is-haptic-feedback/.

D'Arcy, P. (2017, June 7). What the mysterious symbols made by early humans can teach us about how we evolved. https://ideas.ted.com/what-the-mysterious-symbols-made-by-early-humans-can- teach-us-about-how-we-evolved/.

De Luca, R., Leonardi, S., Portaro, S., Le Cause, M., De Domenico, C., Colucci, P. V., Pranio, F., Bramanti, P., & Calabrò, R. S. (2021). Innovative use of virtual reality in autism spectrum disorder: A case-study. *Applied Neuropsychology: Child*, *10*(1), 90–100. https://doi.org/10.1080/21622965.2019.1610964.

Hacmun, I., Regev, D., & Salomon, R. (2018, October 31). The principles of art therapy in virtual reality. *Frontiers in Psychology*. https://doi.org/10.3389/fpsyg.2018.02082.

Kaimal, G., Carroll-Haskins, K., Berberian, M., Dougherty, A., Carlton, N., & Ramakrishnan, A. (2019). Virtual reality in art therapy: A pilot qualitative study of the novel medium and implications for practice. *Art Therapy: Journal of the American Art Therapy Association*, *37*(1), 16–24.

Liu, Y.-C., & Chang, C.-L. (2018). The application of virtual reality technology in art therapy: A case of Tilt Brush. *2018 1st IEEE International Conference on Knowledge Innovation and Invention (ICKII)*, 47–50. https://doi.org/10.1109/ICKII.2018.8569081.

Mesa-Gresa, P., Gil-Gómez, H., Lozano-Quilis, J.-A., & Gil-Gómez, J.-A. (2018). Effectiveness of virtual reality for children and adolescents with Autism Spectrum Disorder: An evidence-based Systematic Review. *Sensors*, *18*(8), 2486. https://doi.org/10.3390/s18082486.

17 Art Therapists and Digital Community

Gretchen M. Miller

Introduction

In the early days of the public's internet use, connecting online with numerous forms of community was a key activity and essential to its emerging practice and purpose (Chen, 2019). A world of potential emerged that was previously unexperienced. Newsgroups, listservs, electronic bulletin boards, and web forums were only some examples of how users could join conversations, exchange information, network, and access content online from around the globe, all from the convenience of a desktop computer.

A small group of innovative art therapists, who started using the Internet during this ground-breaking time, experienced a similar need: to engage in this new technology for connection and community about art therapy and for art therapists (Miller, 2018).

This chapter will begin with an overview of the importance of digital communities for the field of art therapy and touch upon past, present, and an imagining of future developments. Examples will highlight the sustaining impact and implications of digital community for emerging and practicing art therapists, including how the COVID pandemic shed new light and considerations about the necessity of online connection for the field. A time capsule experiment will explore what digital community might look like for art therapists by 2030. With time capsule responses having been collected at the beginning of 2020, some of the predictions have already become reality through the necessities imposed by the COVID pandemic, such as extensive use of videoconferencing to deliver art therapy in a time of social distancing.

History of Digital Community and Art Therapy

Ohler (2010) defines digital communities as "groups to which we belong to that are primarily sustained through electronic rather than geographic proximity" (p. 41). In a digital community, the group and its members can be connected every hour of every day. The first art therapy digital communities emerged as web forums and online networks in the mid-1990s, especially in regions such as the United States, Canada, and the United Kingdom. The

DOI: 10.4324/9781003149538-21

growing use of email and websites provided new possibilities for the field of art therapy to increase communication with colleagues, students, and those interested in learning more about the profession. As a result of the internet's reach, engagement defined by one's geographical and physical location became less necessary to experience worldwide art therapy interaction in the form of collaboration and exchanging information online (Miller, 2018).

The early forms of digital art therapy communities started to further develop with the gradual shift to social networking site activity in the 2000s. A defining characteristic of social media includes its dynamic ability to amplify participation with and connect to one another's user-generated content, widely disseminate, and easily link it to entire communities of social networks and contacts. Social media transformed and activated existing web-based technology into interactive platforms, such as YouTube, Flickr, Blogger, Facebook, Twitter, Instagram, LinkedIn, and Pinterest, where the art therapy community was invited to engage with information in the form of videos, photos, blogs, and social networking to meet other art therapists and students online. The introduction of smartphones created greater access to experience ongoing interaction with online content and virtually connecting to others. Chayko (2014) stated "the ever-increasing use of the Internet, mobile communication, and social media networking catalyzed a revolution in social connectedness [that has been referred to as] the triple revolution" (p. 977).

The foundation built from the community of art therapists who were online in the early days of the internet, supported by the forthcoming presences and popular use of social media in the field, helped develop the global art therapy community to activate a shift in perception to begin crossing what Kapitan described as the "digital culture divide" (2007, p. 50) in our profession. An increase in the application of and value in technology for community and creativity became more visible in the 2010s, as well as becoming more familiar in an art therapist's clinical practice. During this time, I observed an increase in art therapists steadily publishing websites, blogs, podcasts, virtual courses, and sharing personal art and creative practices online, as well as regularly joining art therapy informed digital communities and professional groups on social media.

For example, the discussion and networking groups of the Art Therapy Alliance on LinkedIn, founded in 2008 (https://www.linkedin.com/groups/87161), include a dozen professional communities about art therapy. At the time of writing, this collective network includes over 20,000 users. In 2011, the growing presence of art therapy blog activity inspired the creation of The Art Therapy Blog Index (https://arttherapyalliance.wordpress.com/art-therapy-blog-index). This became an online collection of over 50 art therapy bloggers who submitted their sites to share their experiences as an art therapist or student, their own creative practice, and professional interests in the field.

As our field launches into the decade of 2020 and beyond, the role of digital community has an opportunity for continued growth as a valuable resource to strengthen our collegial relationships, professional work, learning, and cross-cultural connection (Miller, 2018).

Benefits of Digital Community for Art Therapists

Research has documented that relational connection is important to our emotional and physical health and well-being. Forming relationships and being part of a community has been found to reduce isolation, promote resiliency, encourage motivation, manage stress, and create meaningful belonging to others (Martino et al., 2015; Miller, 2016). When individuals are part of a larger community or network, this helps form valuable resources of support, care, and assistance that members have access to and can depend on in times of need. Belonging to a community is a significant need for art therapists professionally, educationally, and artistically. Despite steady growth as a field, art therapists are still from a unique and specialized profession that remains reasonably small in numbers. As of this writing, the Art Therapy Credentials Board (ATCB) in the United States has credentialed over 6,700 art therapists (ATCB, 2021). In comparison, the United States Department of Labor's Bureau of Labor Statistics (2019) cited over 192,000 psychologists, 713,200 social workers, 319,400 mental health counselors, and over 66,000 marriage and family therapists. Art therapists can find great meaning in connecting with others in our field who understand the practice, job, and common challenges. This connection to community provides art therapists with a source of validation, identity, and affinity to our work as clinicians and our creative practice as artists.

Art therapy associations, such as the American Art Therapy Association (AATA), Canadian Art Therapy Association (CATA), and British Association of Art Therapists (BAAT), use online platforms, such as Facebook, LinkedIn, Twitter, and Instagram to not only interact with their members, but also to provide connection, community, and creativity to the greater art therapy field and public at large. For example, in 2018, the AATA launched MyAATA, an online community forum especially for members to "explore, network, and engage with each other and with industry experts" (AATA, 2018). With over 4000 member users and hundreds of contributors, this platform has become an active means of engagement over the last four years for community members to share resources, questions, and dialogue about current topics and interests related to studying and practicing art therapy (AATA, 2021).

Another example is the Art Therapy Students Associated (ATSA), an online group founded in 2020, hosted on Facebook and run by Adler University graduate art therapy students Hannah Tezak, Robert Turk, and Zachary Van Den Berg for students in the art therapy community. The purpose of this digital group is to activate resources for emerging art therapists in the United States and beyond. ATSA aims to promote shared experiences online to mobilize art therapy students and the art therapy community at large around learning, networking, and art-based opportunities to help augment one's educational experience.

In a personal communication in November 2020, Van Den Berg speaks to another advantage of digital communities, which includes embracing an environment based on egalitarian values. Egalitarianism believes that everyone participating in the group is an equal and valuable contributor regardless of differences in status and hierarchical roles (Collie et al., 2017). Online mobilization of resources and collective activity is driven by the ongoing generosity of the group to assist, empower, and support the digital community (Rodgers, 2011). This communal quality is leveraged in the virtual setting, where participation access is easily available to art therapists in comparison to barriers commonly experienced in offline environments. Contributions from all members are viewed as welcomed, significant, and appreciated for the betterment and affirmation of the digital community.

Digital communities also value participatory culture (Humphreys, 2016). The egalitarian nature of the virtual environment encourages art therapists to engage in the free, open, and mutual exchange of ideas, resources, creative expression, and interpersonal connection (Miller, 2018). Collie et al. (2017) highlight that online spaces help equalize differences. In a digital community, this can provide parallel access despite our varying physical locations, educational or professional statuses, and affiliations. Art therapy students, new professionals, practicing art therapists, seasoned experts, and retirees from around the world can collectively access opportunities for online interaction to foster connection in our art therapy work or studies. This engagement can assist in managing stress and coping through finding shared support, professional camaraderie, and resilience together. The equalitarian environment is also experienced by art therapists in artmaking communities hosted online (Gerity, 2010). Community members in these digital spaces find commonality together through creative acts as artists.

Art Therapists and Digital Community During COVID-19

With the onset of the pandemic in early 2020, art therapy students and educators quickly moved to emergency remote learning (American Art Therapy Association, 2020a). Physical interaction and connection experienced extreme limitation and safety adaptations due to social distancing and infection control protocols. Like many others during this time, the art therapy community turned to technology and online connection to cope with this new state of the world we were all living, working, and learning in (Miller & McDonald, 2020).

In response to the evolving situation with COVID-19, I reached out through social media platforms to invite art therapists, students, and other creatives to participate in a community-based Artist Trading Card (ATC) exchange and eventual art mail swap to help manage what we were experiencing. No matter where we each lived, the impact of this pandemic was far reaching in our daily lives, work, studies, relationships, and overall well-being. A virtual community collaboration in our isolated physical creative spaces and home studios offered an opportunity to come together through art making during a time of great uncertainty and distress.

This project included 100 participants from six different countries who signed up to make three handmade and original ATCs in any art media which reflected the exchange's theme of Creative Contact. ATCs are miniature pieces of art about the size of a playing card, 2.5 x 3.5 inches or 64 mm x 89 mm. Participants were invited to reflect on what their own definition or connection to *creative contact* might be, especially in the times of COVID-19. Each participant worked on their ATCs from March through May 2020 with plans that participants would be physically exchanging their images with others in the swap through the postal mail.

Besides creating ATCs on our own during this time, the collaboration used the power of the internet and digital community to help us stay connected throughout the process, which was especially meaningful and valuable during this time of quarantine and separation. This included a digital community hosted through Facebook Groups where participants could share the creative space they were working in during this period of lockdown as well as share their created ATCs with others involved in the exchange (Figures 17.1 and 17.2).

This virtual space encouraged safe ways to gather with others and we supported one another through a stressful situation using our creativity and art making. Other popular social media platforms were also used by participants to share art and communicate experiences using the hashtag #creativecontactATCswap.

Another form of online connection that took place during this project was inviting this participant community to virtually create together during video meetups on Zoom (Figure 17.3). These scheduled times involved moments

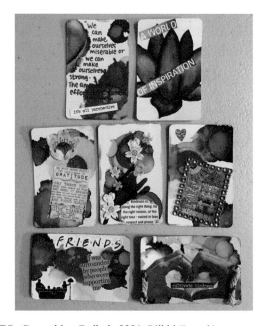

Figure 17.1 ATCs Created by @nikolet2331 (Nikki Fenech)

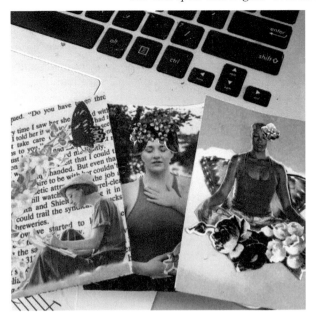

Figure 17.2 ATCs Created By @sjbcreates (Sharon Burton)

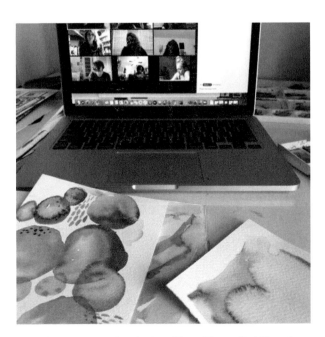

Figure 17.3 Creative Contact Virtual Meet Up – Photo: @phillyarttherapy (Kathryn Snyder)

where we could work on our ATCs together, share what we were making or ideas we had, the art media we were using, how we were coping with COVID-19, and get to know others involved in the exchange. The meetups allowed us an hour or two to be together in creative community while collectively managing such an intense and extreme situation.

The *Art Therapy During A Mental Health Crisis: Coronavirus Pandemic Impact Report* (American Art Therapy Association, 2020b) examined how art therapists were coping with the effects of the pandemic. Anxiety due to social isolation was identified in 61% of respondents. Art therapists also reported relying on self-care with personal art making and belonging to a community as valuable to their own coping throughout the pandemic. "Art was most frequently mentioned when asked, what, if anything, is giving you hope or motivation?" (American Art Therapy Association, 2020b, p. 17).

This was identified as well among many Creative Contact ATC exchange participants. Expression of gratitude, inspiration, and connection was apparent amidst what we were all encountering because of the pandemic's uncertainty and impact. For example, art therapist Kelly Jacobs shared this reflection with her ATCs (see Figure 17.4) in our digital community:

> While creating these I was really thinking about how the changes that we are making right now in the face of the coronavirus could have such potential for positive growth and overall betterment. My creative mind

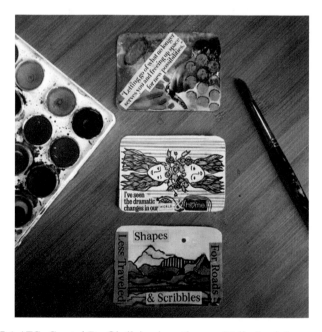

Figure 17.4 ATCs Created By @kellyjacobs.arttherapy (Kelly Jacobs)

has been expanding and exploring all the new possibilities that could emerge from the limitations with which we are now confronted. This art exchange has been one of the bright spots in helping to see the positives!

(K. Jacobs, personal communication, May 11, 2020)

New art therapist Nikki Fenech reached out with this response:

In addition to making the ATCs, this process ignited my creativity and connection to the healing through art process that I lost touch with from not being able to work and dropping the ball on my own self-care… . I was just ready to look for something part-time, gathering letters of reference and updating my resume right before things got bad with the pandemic. Anyway, this group was the first time I've felt like an art therapist since the AATA conference, so thank you.

(N. Fenech, personal communication, May 11, 2020)

After engaging entirely virtually, over 300 ATCs were collectively made and mailed by post a couple of months later. The digital connection and community was now transforming. Each handmade ATC was a physical and in-person connection that could be touched and held by someone in our community, something that takes on new meaning in response to coping with social distancing. ATC mail travelled through several states, regions, and countries before safely arriving in the hands and hearts of each participant (Figure 17.5).

Finally, the report *Art Therapy in Pandemics: Lessons for COVID-19* (Potash et al., 2020) highlighted creative virtual communities as a valuable means to unite shared belonging and increase hope during a time that was marked by separation, detachment, stress, and loss. I believe the circumstances of COVID-19 helped bring a new understanding, validation, and appreciation to the use of digital community not fully experienced before.

The Future of Digital Community for Art Therapists

At the beginning of 2020, I initiated a digital time capsule about technology and art therapy with the intention of responses to be re-visited in 2030 as a fun way to look at how the state of our online and computer-assisted behaviours and activities over a decade may have changed. The time capsule consisted of an online form with 10 questions. The link to the form was distributed to my social media networks over the first month of 2020. Approximately 20 responses were received from art therapists and art therapy students. They provided their thoughts and experiences about existing technology use in 2020, as well as hopes and caution for technology's role in 2030 related to connection and art therapy. It is important to note that many responding to my invitation were already comfortable with using technology in their personal and professional lives, which means collected impressions may not be representative of all art therapists.

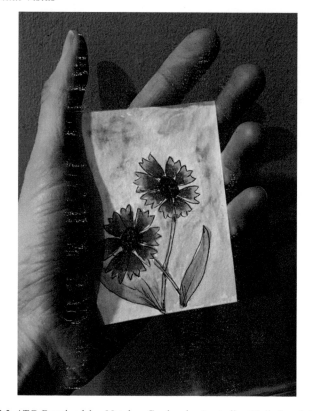

Figure 17.5 ATC Received by Natalya Garden in Australia, Mailed and Created by
@creativityintherapy (Carolyn Stalzer) in United States

What time capsule participants wanted to learn more about in the next
decade included video use, augmented reality, artificial intelligence, and collaborative and integrative virtual art-making. Leveraging technology's portable
nature to make art therapy more available was also noted in responses. Time
capsule contributors envisioned that, by 2030, art therapists may be using
telecommunication technology worldwide as a preferred mode of engagement
to work with clients, expand access, collaborate with colleagues, easily conduct global research and outreach, and democratize information. Furthermore,
virtual technology may become an increasingly familiar environment for
attending conferences and workshops. Participants imagined that virtual reality, new digital applications based on sensory absorbed experiences, and the
use of robots would impact the art therapy community's practice, learning,
education, and access to diverse connections.

Respondents also expressed concerns and cautions about the future, such as
the impact from a lack of in-person contact and a worry that traditional art
making with physical materials in offline spaces may be replaced. Managing

the amount of digital intake we are exposed to, keeping up with the quickening pace of technology, and ethical factors were also included. These considerations have historically been common warnings among art therapists (Klorer, 2009; Miller, 2018), and will continue to have an ongoing presence in some form as the art therapy field keeps moving with technology.

However, there was an overall hopefulness and excitement about the future possibilities of art therapy and technology to strengthen our work as art therapists and as a global profession. By 2030, time capsule responses predicted technology would be commonly used for art therapists to provide intervention from anywhere in the world, counteract community isolation, and maintain meaningful, compassionate digital relational spaces among a hyper techno-connected world in need of refuge and safe haven.

It is noteworthy that responses submitted for this time capsule happened immediately before the COVID-19 pandemic took hold around the world. In a matter of weeks, some of these predictions and reflections about the future of art therapy and technology started to emerge in the field out of necessity to serve clients, students, and communities remotely. For example, participants were invited to share a technology-related skill that they would like to do more with or learn about as an art therapist over the next decade. Digital art programs or apps to use in sessions, making videos, or learning more about the use of distance art therapy, webinars, and art-based technology to increase accessibility and portability were among some interests identified. Due to the impact of COVID-19, these areas of technology experienced an acceleration of engagement in the art therapy community. Videos became a form of remote art therapy (Children's National, 2020), with many art therapy services shifting completely online with new creative approaches and platforms (American Art Therapy Association, 2020b; Miller & McDonald, 2020). Art therapy education was delivered virtually in academic programs (American Art Therapy Association, 2020a). In addition, professional development and collegial connections experienced tremendous growth through virtual membership meetings, online conferences, and webinars since meeting in-person was not advisable due to COVID-19 safety protocols.

Another time capsule consideration voiced was the hope that teletherapy services would become more recognized, available, and respected as an effective treatment option in the next 10 years. In the first few months of 2020, the pandemic pushed many art therapists and art therapy programs to rethink how they could provide services to clients they could no longer see in person because of COVID-19 restrictions. A new awareness and practical curiosity about the benefits and possibilities of teletherapy started to emerge (American Art Therapy Association, 2020b).

Conclusion

Digital community for art therapists retains lasting principles grounded in a rich history of connection and innovation. Virtual engagement within the field continues to forge strong bonds that unite our professional need for belonging, support, and knowledge online. As technology grows and develops, so will art therapy's use of its tools, platforms, and applications for community, engagement, and practice. Art therapists have come a long way from the field's small beginnings and activity online. As the time capsule responses show, the possibilities that lie ahead for digital community will be exciting to witness as art therapists discover and apply new ways for connecting virtually and the impact of this on our practice, creativity, and community.

References

American Art Therapy Association (AATA). (2021). About our members: AATA at a glance 2021. https://arttherapy.org/news-member-infographic.

American Art Therapy Association. (2020a). *To my colleagues that are changing everything, here are 5 tips for effectively teaching art therapy online.* https://arttherapy.org/blog-5-tips-for-teaching-art-therapy-online.

American Art Therapy Association. (2020b). *Art therapy during a mental health crisis: Coronavirus pandemic impact report.* https://arttherapy.org/upload/Art-Therapy-Coronavirus-Impact-Report.pdf.

American Art Therapy Association (AATA). (2018). Save the date: New MyAATA online community opens August 8. https://arttherapy.org/news-myaata-online-member-community-opens-august-8.

Art Therapy Credentials Board (ATCB). (2021). Find a credentialed art therapist. http://www.atcb.org.

Bureau of Labor Statistics, U.S. Department of Labor. (2019). Occupational outlook handbook. https://www.bls.gov/ooh/occupation-finder.htm.

Chayko, M. (2014). Techno-social life: The internet, digital technology, and social connectedness. *Sociology Compass, 8*: 976–991, https://www.doi.org/10.1111/soc4.12190.

Chen, R. (2019). The history of internet communities. [Medium Post]. https://medium.com/@rchen8/the-history-of-internet-communities-f0234db848b1

Children's National. (2020). Remote art therapy resources. https://childrensnational.org/visit/resources-for-families/creative-services/creative-and-therapeutic-arts/art-therapy/remote-art-therapy.

Collie, K., Prins Hankinson, S., Norton, M., Dunlop, C., Mooney, M., Miller, G., & Giese-Davis, J. (2017). Online art therapy groups for young adults with cancer. *Arts & Health, 9*(1), 1–13, https://www.doi.org/10.1080/17533015.2015.1121882.

Gerity, L. (2010). Fourteen secrets for a happy artist's life: Using art and the Internet to encourage resilience, joy, and a sense of community. In C. Hyland Moon (Ed.), *Materials and Media in Art Therapy: Critical Understandings of Diverse Artistic Vocabularies* (pp.155–182). New York, NY: Routledge.

Humphreys, A. (2016). *Social media: Enduring principles.* New York, NY: Oxford University Press.

Kapitan, L. (2007). Will art therapy cross the digital culture divide? *Art Therapy: Journal of the American Art Therapy Association, 24*(2), 50–51. https://www.doi.org/10.1080/07421656.2007.10129591.

Klorer, G. (2009). The effects of technological overload on children: An art therapist's perspective. *Art Therapy: Journal of the American Art Therapy Association, 26*(2), 80–82, https://www.doi.org/10.1080/07421656.2009.10129742.

Martino, J., Pegg, J., & Frates, E. P. (2015). The connection prescription: Using the power of social interactions and the deep desire for connectedness to empower health and wellness. *American Journal of Lifestyle Medicine*, *11*(6), 466–475. https://www.doi.org/10.1177/1559827615608788.

Miller, G. (2016). Social media and creative motivation. In R. Garner (Ed.) *Digital Art Therapy: Material, Methods, and Applications* (pp. 40–53). Philadelphia, PA: Jessica Kingsley Publishers.

Miller, G. (2018). *The art therapist's guide to social media*. New York, NY: Routledge.

Miller, G., & McDonald, A. (2020). Online art therapy during the COVID-19 pandemic. *International Journal of Art Therapy: Inscape*, *25*(4), 159–160, https://www.doi.org/10.1080/17454832.2020.1846383.

Ohler, J. B. (2010). *Digital community, digital citizen*. Thousand Oaks, CA: Corwin.

Potash, J. S., Kalmanowitz, D., Fung, I., Anand, S.A., & Miller, G. M. (2020). Art therapy in pandemics: Lessons for COVID-19. *Art Therapy: Journal of the American Art Therapy Association*, *37*(2), 105–107, https://www.doi.org/10.1080/07421656.2020.1754047.

Rodgers, K.E. (2011). Virtual communities as egalitarian societies: Why contributions matter and what they mean. *Anthropology Department Theses and Dissertations*, *17*. https://digitalcommons.unl.edu/anthrotheses/17.

Index

communication; older adults, and virtual art therapy
virtual art therapy clinic (VATC) 40–50, 112, 174, 178
virtual dynamics 78–80
virtual house call 15
virtual reality (VR) technology, art therapy with: adoption of VR in art therapy 199; as art making tool 197–198; and cognitive behavioural therapy 201–202; limitations 202–205; overview 195–196; visions of future 205–206
virtual space 78–80, 128, 153, 202, 203, 205, 212
virtual studio *see* open studio model in art therapy
virtual supervision 113–115
virtual therapeutic space, navigating 29
virtual touring 49
voice communication without video 18
volunteers, input from 20–21
vulnerability 1, 9, 17, 19, 21, 29, 73, 74

walking studios 151–154
Walls, J. 178, 179
Walther, J. B. 16
Wan, X. 176
Wang, C. 176
Weblogs 13
Web Whiteboard, A (AWW) **56**
Weinberg, H. 171

Weinberg, N. 17
WhatsApp 27
Whitaker, P. 151–152
Whiteboard, Zoom 90, 112, 118, 119, 121, 124
Whiteside, A. 140
Williams, N. 177
Winkel, M. 83–84, 112, 154, 167
World Health Organization 174, 176, 177
World Wide Web 13

Xiao, H. 176
Xu, L. 176

Yang, N. 176
youth: engagement, social media for 29; PYD 65; *see also* Summer Arts Workshop (SAW) in Los Angeles
YouTube 89, 90, 209

Zaylor, C. 3
Zhang, Y. 176
zine project 72, 75
Zoom 2, 15, 67, 68, 69, 72; art therapists during COVID-19 212, *213*, 214; art therapy groups 88–94; fatigue 89; for healthcare 88, 90; studio to chat room to 86–90; Whiteboard 90, 112, 118, 119, 121, 124; *see also* group arts-based therapy via Zoom
Zubala, A. 23, 27

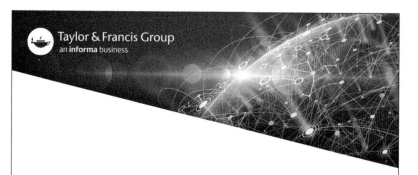

For Product Safety Concerns and Information please contact our
EU representative GPSR@taylorandfrancis.com Taylor & Francis
Verlag GmbH, Kaufingerstraße 24, 80331 München, Germany